HYPERPARATHYROIDISM

Edited by **Gonzalo Díaz-Soto**
and **Manuel Puig-Domingo**

Hyperparathyroidism
Edited by Gonzalo Díaz-Soto and Manuel Puig-Domingo

Published by InTech

Janeza Trdine 9, 51000 Rijeka, Croatia

Publishing Process Manager Romana Vukelic

Technical Editor Teodora Smiljanic

Cover Designer InTech Design Team

Additional hard copies can be obtained from orders@intechopen.com

Hyperparathyroidism, Edited by Gonzalo Díaz-Soto and Manuel Puig-Domingo
p. cm.
ISBN 978-953-51-0478-0

For EU product safety concerns:
IN TECH d.o.o., Prolaz Marije Krucifikse Kozulić 3, 51000 Rijeka, Croatia,
info@intechopen.com or visit our website at intechopen.com.

Meet the editors

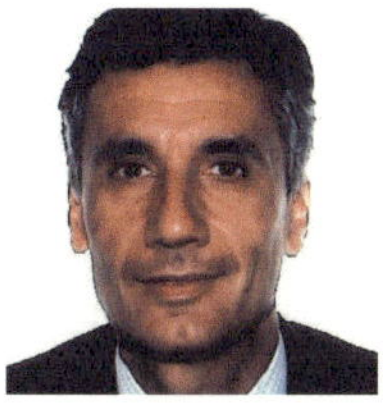

Dr Manuel Puig Domingo is currently Head of the Service of Endocrinology and Nutrition at Germans Trias i Pujol University Hospital and Associate Professor of Endocrinology at the Autonomous University of Barcelona. He received his training in endocrinology and diabetes at Hospital de Sant Pau in Barcelona and a postdoctoral fellowship at the University of Texas in San Antonio. He has been awarded a grant by the Spanish Ministry of Education and has served as an Endocrinologist at Hospital de Sant Pau, Medical Director and Research Director at Hospital de Mataró and Consultant Endocrinologist at Hospital Clínic in Barcelona. Dr Puig has been appointed Vice-President of the Catalan Society of Endocrinology and Nutrition, Vice President of the Spanish Society of Endocrinology and Nutrition, and has also been a member of the directive board of the Spanish Society of Diabetes.

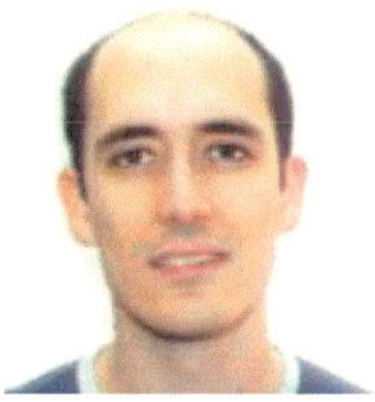

Dr Gonzalo Díaz-Soto is Associate Professor of Endocrinology and Nutrition in Medical School of Valladolid University and researcher at the Endocrinology and Nutrition Institute (IEN) at the same University. He received his MD and Master in Bioscience in experimental Endocrinology on Calcium Sensing Receptor from the Medical School of Valladolid. He finished his specialisation on Endocrinology and Nutrition in the Hospital Clinic of Barcelona. He currently works at the Clinical University Hospital of Valladolid in the Endocrinology, Diabetes and Nutrition Department.

Contents

Preface

Hyperparathyroidism is currently one of the most exciting fields in endocrinology. It is under constant development due to extent of the clinical spectrum of primary hyperparathyroidism. In addition, its relationship with other disorders as secondary/tertiary hyperparathyroidism (mainly in the context of chronic renal failure or haemodialysis) and its complications calls for a particularly complex approach and requires evaluation by many specialists.

In the last decade the progress and development of biochemical assays and new imaging techniques has allowed the diagnosis of unsuspected and asymptomatic disease whose therapeutic approach is still in debate (as normocalcemic hyperparathyroidism).

Finally, the progress on minimally invasive parathyroidectomy, intraoperative PTH and radio-guided surgery is changing the paradigm in treatment of hyperparathyroidism.

All these hot spots in endocrinology are addressed in the book that now we present.

This book is the result of the collaboration between worldwide authorities of different specialities and we are grateful to them for the quality of the contributions. The book aims to provide a general but deep view of primary/secondary and tertiary hyperparathyroidism, from a physiological basis to hyperparathyroidism in hemodialyzed patients, as well as new treatment approaches, techniques and surgical scenarios.

We hope that the medical and paramedical researchers will find this book helpful and stimulating. We look forward to sharing knowledge of hyperparathyroidism with a wider audience.

Professor Dr Manuel Puig-Domingo
University Autonoma of Barcelona Medical School, Germans Trias i Pujol, Badalona
Spain

Dr Gonzalo Díaz-Soto
University of Valladolid Medical School, Clinic Hospital, Valladolid
Spain

Part 1

New Trends in Medical Monitoring of Hyperparathyroidism

1

Normocalcemic Primary Hyperparathyroidism

Maria-Teresa Julián[1], Izaskun Olaizola[1],
Gonzalo Díaz-Soto[2] and Manuel Puig-Domingo[1]
[1]*Services of Endocrinology and Nutrition*
Universitary Hospital Germans Trias Pujol., Badalona (Barcelona),
[2]*Clinical and Universitary Hospital of Valladolid, IEN-Valladolid University,*
Spain

1. Introduction

Normocalcemic primary hyperparathyroidism is a new entity which possibly represents a fruste form of the classic clinically symptomatic disease and which has generated a considerable scientific interest in the last decade. Its official recognition is just as recent as in 2008, when an international conference took place for clarifying its nature and relevance (Bilezikian et al., 2009). Its true prevalence is mostly unknown although it is clear that it is recognized more and more in different clinical settings, from internal medicine outpatient clinics to endocrine or rheumatologists consultations. It is a challenging situation for either the clinician and the patient, as therapeutic recommendations are nowadays nor established and different patients may be advised to receive certain active treatment or just follow-up, or even no follow-up. In this chapter the current data in relation to this emergent condition are presented.

2. Definition and biochemical considerations

Normocalcemic primary hyperparathyroidism (NPHPT) is defined by a situation in which persistently normal serum calcium levels are observed in the presence of high levels of parathyroid hormone (PTH). The term normocalcemic primary hyperparathyroidism was first used in the decade of the 60's by Wills (Wills et al., 1967), who described a group of patients with characteristics different from those with classic primary hyperparathyroidism in which the patients presented a paucity of clinical symptoms and signs and hypercalcemia was absent. No other terms have been used, such as subclinical hyperparathyroidism or low grade primary hyperparathyroidism have been used in the definition of this condition, as it has been the case for similar endocrine disturbances like i.e. subclinical hypothyroidism. The definition of normocalcemic primary HPT' includes total albumin-corrected serum calcium within the normal range and serum parathyroid hormone (PTH) relatively elevated in comparison to the serum calcium level.

Under such a biological combination a search for causes that may reveal a secondary hyperparathyroidism syndrome is the first step that the clinician uses to face, and mostly all situations that could favor vitamin D deficiency, a condition very prevalent all over the world (Silverberg et al., 2009), need to be ruled out. In fact this is a major problem, as in most cases it is not known if the reference range of a given PTH assay has been made with a population in which vitamin D deficiency exclusion criteria has been considered. PTH is a heterogeneous molecule, and in the last 25 years its measurement has been performed with different assays which have been experimented technological evolution. We have been using different generations of assays and currently we under in the third generation era; the sensitivity of second- and third generation PTH assays in detecting elevated PTH values seems to be similar (Eastell R et al., 2009). By using a second-generation PTH assay it has been recognized how important it is to exclude subjects with low serum 25OHD levels in establishing a reference range for PTH (Souberbielle JC et al., 2001). When this is taken into account, the upper limit of the PTH reference interval for second-generation assays decreased from 65 to 46 ng/liter, a 29% reduction. The same applies for establishing a reference interval for "whole PTH" assays the upper limit decreasing from 44 to 34 ng/L, a 27% reduction; finally, the upper limit of the reference interval remains also lower for third generation assays than for second-generation ones. It has to be mentioned that in parallel, vitamin D references values have been established in the last decades, and moreover, there is still a debate going on in relation to what are the lower normal values (Looker et al., 2008). In some studies, values below 20 ng/mL were taken as the lower limit of vitamin D sufficiency, whereas other studies have reported that PTH levels in normocalcemic individuals continue to decline until levels of 25OHD above 30 ng/ml have been achieved (Chapuy et al., 1992, 2002; Dawson-Hughes et al., 1997). This emphasizes the importance of establishing an international consensus on a reference range for 25OHD, if we are to improve the reference range of PTH by excluding subjects with vitamin D insufficiency. A very interesting approach has been recently proposed by Harvey et al (Harvey A et al., 2011), by using a nomogram in which vitamin D and age are included for refining the diagnosis of primary hyperparathyroidism.

3. Epidemiology

There is virtually no data in relation to the epidemiology of NPHPT. Lundgren and cols. (Lundgren E et al., 2002; Tordjman et al., 2004) studied more than 5,000 postmenopausal women between the ages of 55 and 75 in Swedish survey. They found that 16% of individuals had normal serum calcium levels (< 9.9 mg/dL) and elevated PTH. This group included both those with vitamin D deficiency which was not ruled out and non-deficient cases which could effectively considered as the true cases of normocalcemic PHPT. Taken together both situations, the prevalence seems really surprising and thus will imply that this disorder is the most prevalent endocrine disorder so far. More data are warranted in order to confirm such a potential high prevalence.

4. Clinical presentation

It is not known if NPHPT is an indolent disease or if it may have an impact similar, to certain extent, to the classic primary hyperparathyroidism bone metabolism dysfunction and renal damage as a consequence of sustained circulating increased PTH. It is also not known if increased PTH per se may have pathological consequences as the disorder goes on –if it would be true that progression is universal in all cases- and if therapeutic intervention aimed to normalize PTH may have any benefit at short and long term in these patients. Therefore it is very important to conduct studies in order to clarify all this lack of information.

Usually, NPHPT is discovered in the context of an evaluation of patients with low bone density in specialized metabolic bone units, in whom secondary causes for increased PTH concentration have been carefully ruled out. However, some patients can present with some clinical features of classical hyperparathyroidism, such as fragility fracture and kidney stones. Lowe et al. (Lowe et al., 2007) evaluated thirty-seven patients who met criteria of NPHPT. At the moment of presentation, 14% of the patients had a history of nephrolithiasis and 46 % had a history of fracture in adulthood. Bone mineral density assessment showed that 57% had osteoporosis in at least one site (lumbar-spine, hip or distal radius), 19% had osteoporosis at two of three sites and 8% were osteoporotic at all three sites. Osteoporosis was more common at the lumbar spine (34%) and hip (38%) than in the distal radius (28%), in contrast to the hypercalcemic form of hyperparathyroidism, where preponderance of bone density loss more at the cortical radius site is observed.

There are few studies that evaluated the evolution of this entity at long term. These patients are at some risk of disease progression, further developing features of classical hyperparathyroidism in certain cases. Also, some of these patients will become hypercalcemic over time, and it is observed that those with the higher serum calcium average concentrations and those who were somewhat older were more likely to develop hypercalcemia. On the other hand, some of these patients will suffer from kidney stones, decline in BMD, osteoporosis, and even fractures.

In the cohort of Lowe et al. (Lowe et al., 2007) 41% of the patients showed evidence for progressive hyperparathyroid disease at a median follow up of 3 years: 19% became hypercalcemic, 3% presented kidney stones, 29 % presented progressive cortical bone loss (occurring at all sites) and decline of BMD greater than 10% in 16%; 11% presented new osteoporotic lesions and 3% bone fracture. But on the other side, they also observed that some of the patients with the longest follow up (8 years) did not show evidence of disease progression and may never develop the more typical hypercalcemic phenotype of the disease. Therefore, in some patients there is a progression of the disease and in some other not, and until now there is no way to segregate both cohorts and prediction of progression is not currently feasible.

Overt primary hyperparathyroidism is associated with an increased frequency of dyslipidemia, hypertension, overweight and impaired glucose tolerance. It remains unclear whether NPHPT goes together with such cardiovascular risk factors seen in a much active hyperparathyroid situation when circulating calcium is high. There is very few information in NPHPT and in the only study performed so far (Hagström et al., 2006) some degree of relationship seems to exist although vitamin D deficiency was not assessed in this cohort and it is very well known how important vitamin D sufficiency for cardiovascular protection is (Adams & Hewison., 2010). The relevance of this latter study (Hagström et al., 2006) is that is was performed in general population, while most of the data of NPHPT have been obtained in subjects which have received medical attention mostly because of bone or kidney problems, implying a bias in the interpretation of the non symptomatic nature of this entity.

NPHPT has a pleiotropic phenotypic presentation and nowadays it remains unclear whether it could be the initial phase or and indolent form of classic hyperparathyroidism. Data suggest that it is not the early stage of mild asymptomatic hyperparathyroidism but it could be the earliest form of symptomatic hyperparathyroidism, where the patients have already developed some signs and symptoms of the disease but show normal serum calcium concentration, suggesting that this entity may not be as indolent as previously though.

5. Treatment of asymptomatic HPT

Currently there are no guidelines for the management of NPHPT. Even asymptomatic HPT (defined as hyperparathyroidism that lacks specific symptoms or signs traditionally associated with hypercalcemia) treatment is a controversial subject. Third Workshop on the Management of Asymptomatic Primary Hyperparathyroidism in 2009 tried to clarify surgical/medical versus follow up management depending on severity of the manifestations of disease and age of the patient (Bilezikian et al, 2009).

From First Workshop on the Management of Asymptomatic Primary Hyperparathyroidism in 1990 to present time surgical indications have been changing to an earlier parathyroid surgery (Table 1).

	1990	2002	2008
Serum Calcium (>upper limit of normal)	1-1.6 mg/dl (0.25-0.4 mmol/l)	1.0 mg/dl (0.25 mmol/l)	1.0 mg/dl (0.25 mmol/l)
24 h urinary for calcium	>400 mg/d (>10 mmol/d)	>400 mg/d (>10 mmol/d)	Not recommended
Creatinine clearance (calculated)	Reduced 30%	Reduced 30%	Reduced to < 60 ml/min
BMD	Z-score < -2.0 in forearm	T score <-2.5 at any site	T score <-2.5 at any site and/or previous fracture fragility
Age (year)	<50	<50	<50

Table 1. Evolution of guidelines recommendations for parathyroid surgery in asymptomatic HPT (Bilezikian et al, 2009)

However, pharmacologic approach to management of asymptomatic HPT (selected estrogen receptor modulators, biphosphonates and calcimimetics) is limited to patients in whom surgical treatment is not possible mostly because of surgical risk but in whom serum calcium levels or BMD should be treated.

Anyway, Third Workshop concluded that although surgery is an attractive and definitive choice it is also recognized that medical management can be appropriate in those who do not meet surgical indications or are unable or unwilling to proceed with parathyroidectomy. For those cases, follow-up is adviced by Third Workshop (table 2)

	1990	2002	2008
Serum Calcium	Biannually	Biannually	Annually
24 h urinary calcium	Annually	Not recommended	Not recommended
Creatinine clearance (24 h collections)	Annually	Not recommended	Not recommended
Serum creatinine	Annually	Annually	Annually
Bone density	Annually (forearm)	Annually (3 sites)	Every 1-2 years (3 sites)
Abdominal X ray (ultrasound)	Annually	Not recommended	Not recommended

Table 2. Evolution of management guidelines for patients with asymptomatic primary hyperparathyroidism who do not undergo parathyroidectomy. (Bilezikian et al, 2009)

5.1.1 Surgical treatment of asymptomatic HPT

Current guidelines to surgical management of Asymptomatic HPT include (Table 1) (Udelsman et al, 2009):

1. Serum calcium threshold 1 mg/dl (0.25 mM/liter) above the upper limits of normal range.
2. Peri - Postmenopausal men and women older than 50, with T score of 2.5 or less at the lumbar spine, femoral neck, total hip, or 33% (one third) radius. In premenopausal women and in men younger than 50, the Z-score of 2.5 or less is recommended as the cutpoint.
3. Age less than 50 years old
4. A GFR less than 60ml/min.1.73m2 defined a stage 3 level of renal insufficiency according to the K/DOQI guidelines.

As main change with other consensus statement hypercalciuria in the absence of renal stones or nephrolithiasis, is no longer regarded as an indication for parathyroid surgery as it presence without any other factors has not been established as a kidney stone risk factor.

Asymptomatic HPT has been related to neurocognitive compromise, bone density and fracture risk, nephrolitiasis, even with cardiovascular risk and survival. Unfortunately, the scientific evidence in this area is low. Clinical trials are needed to demonstrate the improvements in these parameters after parathyroidectomy.

Surgical experience is the main variable to avoid surgery complications in parathyroidectomy, Therefore number of cases per year is the most important predictor of clinical outcomes. The type of operative procedure and the employment of operative adjuncts is highly institution specific and should be based on the expertise and resource availability of the surgeon and institution.

Localization techniques of enlarged parathyroid gland (sestamibi scan, CT scan, MRI, between others) have a secondary role on parathyroid surgery and it is confined to localization assistance, never for diagnosis purpose.

99mTC-Sestamibi is probably the most used and sensitive probe to parathyroid localization. Its main characteristic is the capacity of diagnosis of ectopic parathyroid glands and functional information. Neck ultrasound plays a principal role on thyroid nodule and parathyroid gland enlargement evaluation but it is highly dependent on experience and interest of the radiologist performing the study (Soto Gd et al, 2010). Combination of both non invasive techniques as complementary methods are highly recommended because of its safety and sensitive.

In special circumstances other imaging techniques could be of interest (CT scan, MRI, PET scan); even, invasive procedures as parathyroid fine needle aspiration and arteriography and selective venous sampling for PTH. However, all these procedures are expensive, time consuming, and with limited but not negligible risks. Actually, its used is limited to minimally invasive surgery where localization parathyroid gland is essential and in those cases without information in conventional techniques (Udelsman et al, 2009).

5.1.2 Medical treatment of asymptomatic HPT

To the date, pharmacologic approach to management of asymptomatic HPT is limited to patients in whom surgical treatment is not possible because of surgical risk but in whom serum calcium levels or BMD should be treated.

Selective estrogen receptor modulators and bisphosphonates could be of interest in Asymptomatic HPT treatment because of potential BMD increase and fracture risk reduction. Unfortunatelly, none of this treatment have been evaluated in clinical assays neither in hyperparathyroidism nor HPHPT (Khan et al, 2009). Only alendronate treatment was shown to improve BMD in lumbar spine of patients with primary hyperparthyroidism without changes in calcium levels to a degree comparable both to their effects in eucalcemic populations (Khan et al, 2004) What is more, fracture outcome date are not available until now with any of the treatments evaluated.

Calcimimetics is a new pharmacology class that acts as an allosteric modulator of the calcium sensing receptor (CASR) acting to sensitize this receptor to the extracellular calcium. Cinacalcet has been shown to be effective in reducing or normalizing serum calcium levels in several groups of patients with primary hyperparathyroidism with slightly reduces PTH levels and no effects on bone mineral density (Peacock et al, 2005 & Marcocci et al, 2011). Unfortunatelly, there are no data as to whether long term treatment with cinacalcet can prevent the complications of PHPT.

At present, medical treatment is limited for those individuals with Asymptomatic HPT who are unable to undergo corrective surgery for whom skeleton protection is the primary reason for intervention (biphosphonates) or control of serum calcium levels are required (cinacalcet). Further investigation is required in this field

6. Conclusion

Normocalcemic primary hyperparathyroidism is a new entity which possibly represents a fruste form of the classic clinically symptomatic disease and which has generated a considerable scientific interest in the last decade. It is a challenging situation for either the clinician and the patient, as therapeutic recommendations are nowadays nor established and different patients may be advised to receive certain active treatment or just follow-up, or even no follow-up. Further investigation is required to select the best treatment for each patient.

7. References

Adams, JS & Hewison, M. Update in vitamin D. (2010). J Clin Endocrinol Metab, Vol.95; No. 2, pp. 471-478, ISSN 0021-972X.

Bilezikian, JP.; Khan, A. & Potts, JT. (2009). Guidelines for the management of asymptomatic primary hyperparathyroidism: summary statement from the third international workshop. J Clin Endocrinol Metab, Vol.94; No. 2, pp. 335–339, ISSN 0021-972X.

Chapuy, MC.; Arlot, ME.; Duboeuf, F.; Brun, J.; Crouzet, B.; Arnaud, S.; Delmas, PD. & Meunier, PJ. (1992). Vitamin D3 and calcium to prevent hip fractures in the elderly women. N Engl J Med, Vol. 327, No. 23, pp. 1637–1642.

Chapuy, MC.; Pamphile, R.; Paris, E.; Kempf, C.; Schlichting, M.; Arnaud, S.; Garnero, P. & Meunier, PJ. (2002). Combined calcium and vitaminD3 supplementation in elderly women: confirmation of reversal of secondary hyperparathyroidism and hip fracture risk: the Decalyos II study. Osteoporos Int ,Vol.13, No.3, pp.257–264.

Dawson-Hughes, B.; Harris, SS.; Krall, EA. & Dallal,GE. (1997). Effect of calcium and vitamin supplementation on bone density in men and women 65 years of age or older. N Engl J Med, Vol. 337, No. 10, pp.670–676.

Eastell, R.; Arnold, A.; Brandi, ML.; Brown, EM.; D'Amour, P.; Hanley, DA.; Sudhaker-Rao, D.; Rubin, MR.; Goltzman, D.; Silverberg, SJ.; Marx, SJ.; Peacock, M.; Mosekilde, L.; Bouillon, R.& Lewiecki, EM. (2009). Diagnosis of Asymptomatic Primary Hyperparathyroidism: Proceedings of the Third International Workshop. J Clin Endocrinol Metab, Vol 94, No. 2, pp. 340–350, ISSN 0021-972X.

Harvey, A.; Hu, M.; Gupta, M.;Butler, R.; Mitchell, J.; Berber, E.; Siperstein, A. & Milas, M. (2011). A New, Vitamin D- Based, Multidimensional Nomogram for the Diagnosis of Primary Hyperparathyroidism. Endocrine Practice, Vol. 8; pp. 1-21. [Epub ahead of print].

Hagström, E.; Lundgren, E.; Rastad, J. & Hellm, P. (2006). Metabolic abnormalities in patients with normocalcemia hyperparathyroidism detected at a population-based screening. European Journal of Endocrinology, Vol. 155, pp. 33-39, ISSN 0804-4643.

Khan AA, Bilezikian JP & Kung AW (2004). Aleudronate in primary hyperparathyroidism: a doubleblind, randomized, placebo-controlled trial. J Clin Endocrinol Metab. Vol. 89. pp.3319–3325.

Khan AA, Bilezikian JP, & Potts JJ (2009) Asymptomatic primary hyperparathyroidism: a Commentary on the revised guidelines. Endocr pract.Vol. 15 No. 5. pp.494–498.

Looker, AC.; Pfeiffer, CM.; Lacher, DA.; Schleicher, RL.; Picciano, MF. & Yetley, EA. (2008). Serum 25-hydroxyvitamin D status of the US population: 1988-1994 compared with 2000-2004. Am J Clin Nutr, Vol.88, No. 6, pp. 1519-1527.

Lowe, H.; McMahon, DJ.; Rubin, MR.; Bilezikian, JP. & Silverberg, SJ. (2007). Normocalcemic primary hyperparathyroidism: further characterization of a new clinical phenotype. J Clin Endocrinol Metab, Vol.92, No.8, pp. 3001-3005, ISSN 0021-972X.

Lundgren, E.; Hagstrom, EG.; Lundin, J.; Winnerback, MB.; Roos, J.; Ljunghall, S. & Rastad,J. (2002). Primary hyperparathyroidism revisited in menopausal women with serum calcium in the upper normal range at population based screening 8 yrs ago. World J Surg, Vol.226, No. 8, pp.931–936, ISSN 00268-002-6621-0.

Marcocci C & Cetani F. (2011) Update on the use of cinacalcet in the management of primary hyperparathyroidism. Endocrinol Invest. Vol. 21.

Peacock M, Bilezikian JP, Klassen PS, Guo MD, Turner SA, Shoback DM. (2005) Cinacalcethydrochloride maintains long-term normocalcemia in patients with primary hyperparathyroidism. J Clin Endocrinol Metab. Vol. 90. Pp. 135–141.

Tordjman, KM.; Greenman ,Y.; Osher, E.; Shenkerman, G. & Sern, N. (2004). Characterization of normocalcemic primary hyperparathyroidism. Am J Med, Vol. 117, No.11, pp. 861–863.

Silverberg, SJ.; Lewiecki, EM.; Mosekilde, L.; Peacock, M. & Rubin, MR. (2009). Presentation of asymptomatic primary hyperparathyroidism: proceedings of the third international workshop. J Clin Endocrinol Metab, Vol. 94, No.2, pp.351-365, ISSN 0021-972X.

Soto GD, Halperin I, Squarcia M, Lomeña F & Domingo MP (2010) Update in thyroid imaging. The expanding world of thyroid imaging and its translation to clinical practice. Hormones (Athens). Vol. 9 No. 4, pp.287-98.

Souberbielle, JC.; Cormier, C.; Kindermans, C.; Gao, P.; Cantor, T.; Forette. F. & Baulieu, EE. (2001). Vitamin D status and redefining serum parathyroid hormone reference range in the elderly. J Clin Endocrinol Metab, Vol. 86, No.7, pp. 3086–3090, ISSN 0021-972X.

Udelsman R, Pasieka JL, Sturgeon C,Young JEM, & Clark OH Surgery for Asymptomatic Primary Hyperparathyroidism: Proceedings of the Third International Workshop J Clin Endocrinol Metab.Vol.94. No2 pp366–372

Wills, MR.;Pak, CY.; Hammond, WG. & Bartter, FC. (1967). Normocalcemic primary hyperparathyroidism. Am J Med, Vol.47, No. 7, pp.384–91.

Part 2

New Trends in Surgical Treatment on Hyperparathyroidism

2

Parathyroid Adenoma Completely Impacted Within the Thyroid: A Case Report and Literature Review

Yuko Tanaka[1*], Hisato Hara[1] and Yuzuru Kondo[2]
[1]*Department of Breast, Thyroid and Endocrine Surgery, Tsukuba University*
[2]*Department of Pathology, Tsukuba University*
Tennodai, Tsukuba, Ibaraki
Japan

1. Introduction

Primary hyperparathyroidism (PHPT) is the most common cause of hypercalcemia, causing oversecretion of parathyroid hormone from adenomas, hyperplasias or carcinomas. Enlarged parathyroid glands are usually detected by ultrasonography or scintigraphy. After making a diagnosis based on laboratory examinations and imaging studies, the patients with PHPT can be easily treated with surgery to remove the enlarged gland, and 95% of such operations are curative (1-3).

However, we sometimes encounter enlarged parathyroid glands located in uncommon regions, such as within the thyroid, in the thymus, in the mediastinum, in the posterior cervical triangle or in other locations, making it hard to detect the parathyroid.

We recently experienced a case of PHPT whose parathyroid adenoma was completely impacted within the thyroid. Based on the sonographic and scintigraphic features of the lesion, the size and location of the parathyroid gland could be estimated before the surgery. We have also established a hypothesis for how some of the parathyroid glands become located in uncommon regions.

This chapter describes uncommon locations of parathyroid adenoma, particularly within the thyroid. We also report a case and review the pertinent literature regarding its generation.

2. Case presentation

A 58-year-old female underwent surgery for breast cancer a year prior to her current presentation. After the operation, she had received chemotherapy with anthracycline for three months and radiotherapy for one and a half months. After these treatments, she had not been on any medications, such as anti-cancer agents or hormone therapy. The laboratory examination during her first annual check-up after the surgery revealed a high corrected serum calcium level of 11.4 mg/dl. Additional laboratory parameters showed high serum

---

* Corresponding Author

intact parathyroid hormone (iPTH) of 114 pg/ml. Her serum alkaline phosphatase level, 332 U/l, was within the normal limits. She was suspected to have hyperparathyroidism.

She had experienced two pregnancies and delivered twice. Her family history revealed no parathyroid disease, other endocrine disease, nor any malignancies. She had not received radiation to the head and neck area during childhood. She had no complaints such as a loss of appetite, nausea, vomiting, constipation, confusion or impaired thinking and memory, feelings of weakness, fatigue, depression, nor aches and pains. Objectively, neither symptoms of bone thinnings nor kidney srones were present.

Ultrasonography revealed a solid and isoechoic mass, 6.0 x 12.7 x 9.8 mm in size, with a regular shape and contour in the middle of the right lobe of the thyroid. The tumor showed a homogeneous internal echo with a high degree of Doppler signaling and was completely embedded in the thyroid, thus suggesting a thyroid tumor (Figure 1a). A technetium-99m MIBI scintigram demonstrated a focal accumulation in the middle of the right lobe of the thyroid from the early phase to the delayed phase (Figure 1b). These findings suggested that the right lower parathyroid gland might be morbid and it could be inside the thyroid parenchyma.

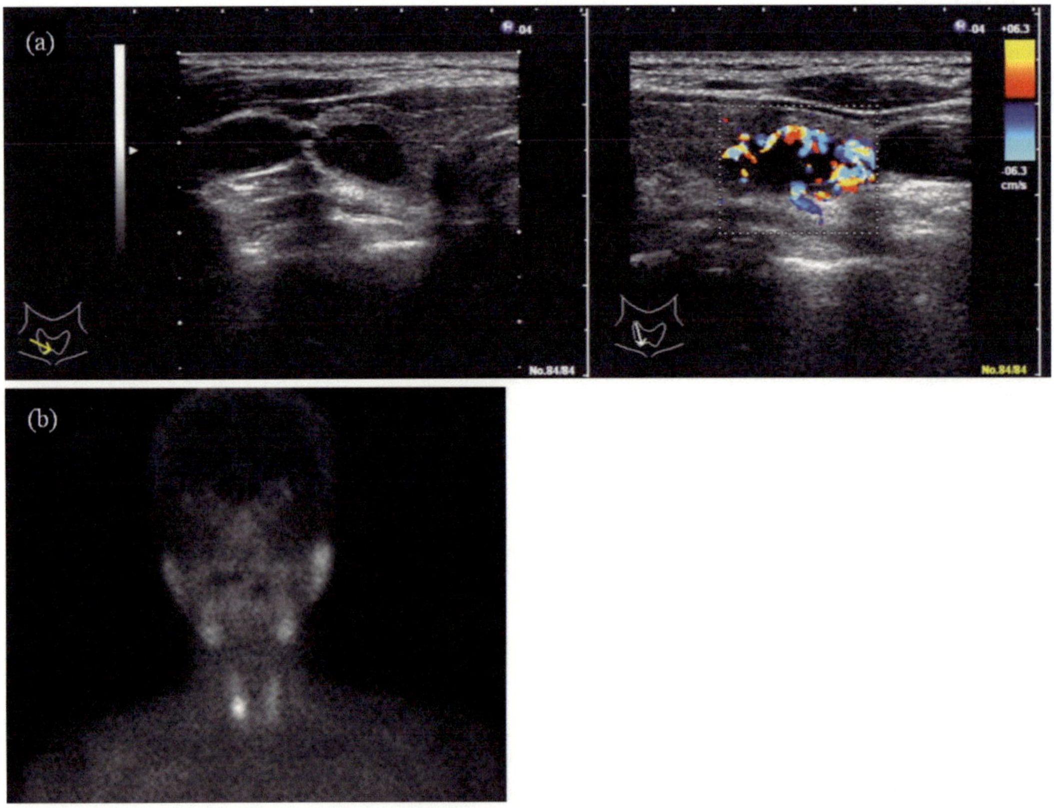

Fig. 1. a) Ultrasonography of the right lobe of the thyroid showing a hypoechoic and hypervascular Doppler signaling mass impacted within the thyroid.
b) A technetium-99m MIBI scintigram demonstrated a focal accumulation in the middle-lower part of the right lobe of the thyroid.

We diagnosed the patient with asymptomatic PHPT and predicted that its location was in the right lobe of the thyroid. The observations during the surgery revealed a morbid parathyroid gland as predicted. It was completely impacted within the right lobe of the thyroid. A right lobectomy of the thyroid was performed, and the right upper parathyroid gland was also removed. The right upper gland located at the cricothyroidal junction was normal.

The histopathological findings of the specimen were as follows: A tumor measuring 9 x 6 x 5 mm in size was located in the middle portion of the right lobe (Figure 2a). The enlarged parathyroid gland had proliferated, displacing the thyroid parenchyma. Microscopically, fat was displaced by the proliferation of chief cells with pale clear cytoplasm arranged in sheets in a solid-alveolar or sinusoidal pattern. Deposits of hemosiderin and cystic changes were also present in the tumor. Mitoses were difficult to detect. All of the tumor cells remained within a fibrous capsule that surrounded the tumor, without direct invasion to the thyroid parenchyma. No capsular or vascular invasion was observed (Figure 2b). The right upper parathyroid and the thyroid parenchyma showed no abnormal findings. The diagnosis was adenoma of the right lower parathyroid gland.

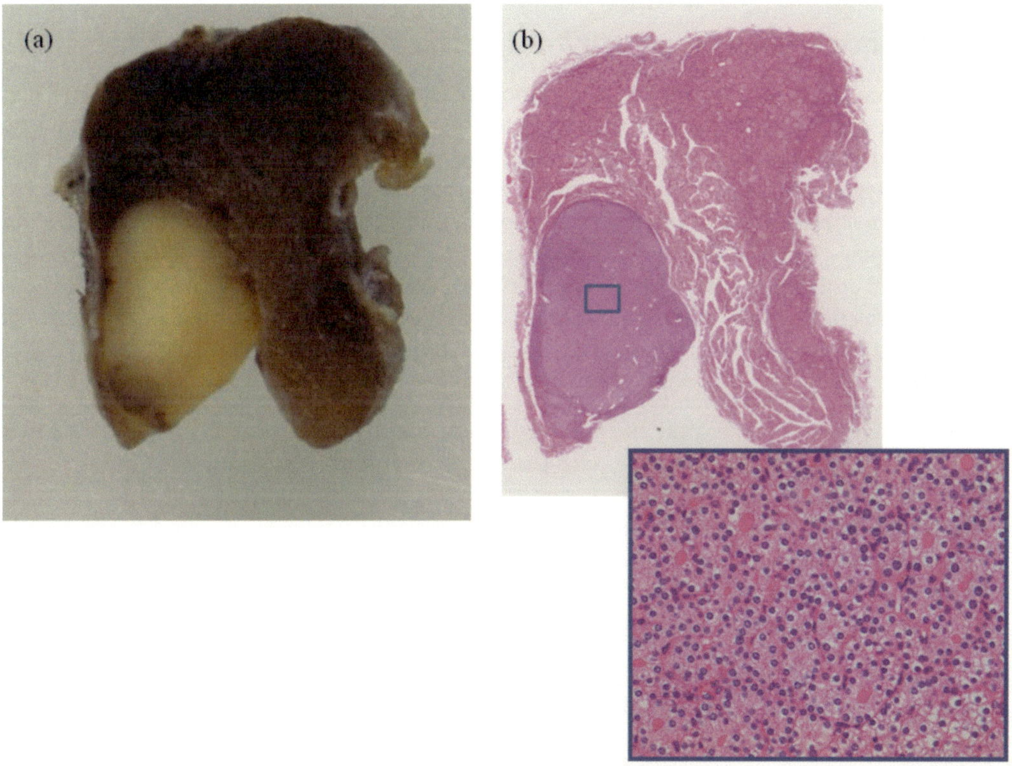

Fig. 2. a) Macroscopic appearance of the specimen showing a tumor measuring 9 x 6 x 5 mm in size located in the middle portion of the right lobe of the thyroid.
b) Microscopic appearance of the tumor diagnosed as parathyroid adenoma, showing the proliferation of chief cells with pale clear cytoplasm arranged in sheets in a solid-alveolar or sinusoidal pattern without mitoses.

There were no complications due to the surgery. After the operation, her serum calcium and iPTH levels were maintained within the normal limits.

3. Parathyroid glands

There are four parathyroid glands, with average weights of 30-40 mg, although the weights vary somewhat with age and sex. Since the glands are soft and pliable in consistency, they are easily shaped and molded by the adjacent tissue. The consistency of morbid parathyroid glands varies (4). In case of adenoma and hyperplasia, accounting for more 85-% of PHPT, the parathyroid glands are relatively hard compared to the normal glands, although they are generally as soft as the thyroid parenchyma. In cases of parathyroid carcinoma, accounting for 1-% to 5-% of PHPT (5), the glands are elastic and hard, which facilitates the diagnosis before and during the operation. Although it can be difficult, we try to make a differential diagnosis between benign and malignant parathyroid disease using real-time tissue elastography before surgery. Elastography shows that the parathyroid carcinomas are definitely harder than the thyroid parenchyma, whereas the adenomas and hyperplasia are as soft as the thyroid parenchyma (Figure 3).

4. Common locations of the parathyroid glands

The expected locations of the parathyroid glands are behind the thyroid parenchyma. They adhere behind the thyroid parenchyma on the bilateral, upper and lower sides of the thyroid. The upper parathyroid glands are located one-third or halfway from the upper poles of the thyroid, and 80-% of the upper parathyroid glands are located within 1 cm around the 1 cm caudal portion from the crossing point of the recurrent laryngeal nerve and the inferior thyroid artery. They sometimes seem to float within the cyst in the thyroid capsule around the upper border of the cricoid cartilage, or posteriorly around the cricothyroid junction. The glands are often intimately associated with the recurrent laryngeal nerve and adjacent vascular branches.

The lower glands are more widely distributed than the upper glands. These glands are distributed between the lower pole of the thyroid and the thymus. It has been estimated that 95-% of the lower glands are located within a 2 cm region around the lower poles of the thyroid. They are found in the anterior or lateroposterior surface of the thyroid. Approximately 40-60-% of the glands adhere to the thyroid parenchyma, and these glands are frequently hidden between the thyroid creases, with 25-40-% being located within the neck of the thymus. They are commonly located in front of the recurrent laryngeal nerves.

Although almost all the parathyroid glands on each side, 80-90-% of the upper glands and 64-70-% of the lower glands are located symmetrically, however, the left parathyroid glands are occasionally located somewhat inferior to the right glands (4, 6).

5. Uncommon locations of the parathyroid glands

a. On the basis of embryological development

The parathyroid glands begin to form from the epithelium of the third and fourth pharyngeal pouches. The upper glands begin in the fourth pouch, and fall back to the upper one-third of the thyroid. If the upper gland lies in an athypical location, it will generally be

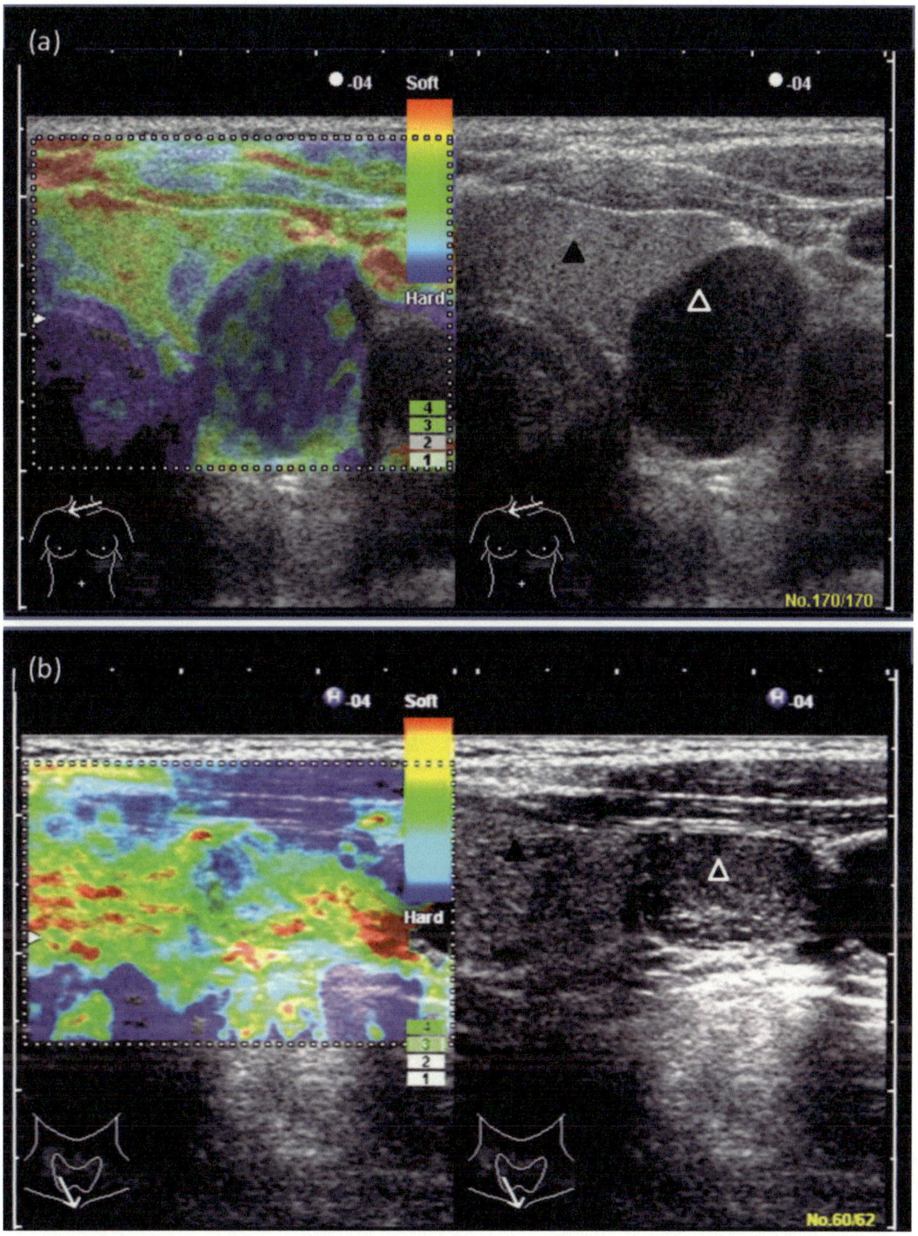

Fig. 3. (a) Elastography of the parathyroid carcinoma showing hard elasticity of the mass
(b) Elastography of the parathyroid hyperplasia showing soft elasticity of the mass
(▲; thyroid parenchyma. △; parathyroid gland)

found in the back of the upper pole of the thyroid, rarely below the lower thyroid artery, and extremely rarely above of the thyroid pole, retropharyngoesophagus space, or in the thyroid parenchyma.

The lower parathyroid glands and thymus begin from the epithelium of the third pharyngeal pouch. As a complex, they descend caudally through the lateral side of the thyroid. They separate, and then the lower parathyroid gland dissociates from thymus and localizes to the anterior or lateroposterior aspect of the lower thyroid pole, and the thymus localizes inside of the mediastinal space. Since the lower glands descend a long distance, there are frequent positional aberrations. For example, if they never descend, they lie in the submandibular space on the lateral side of the common carotid artery and the internal jugular vein, the so-called lateral triangle, or within the carotid sheath. If they descend incompletely, they are called an "undescended parathymus". If they do not separate, the parathyroid glands descend with the thymus into the mediastinum, or may be left high in the neck as a result of early developmental arrest. In nearly half of the cases, the lower gland remains within the thymic tongue at the thoracic inlet. Thus, the lower gland may be found anywhere from the angle of the jaw to the pericardium. Some rare reports have demonstrated even more unusual locations for the parathyroid gland, such as on the base of the heart, in the front of the heart sac, and in the aorto-pulmonary window (4).

b. The cases where enlarged parathyroid glands descend due to of the effects of gravity

Although parathyroid carcinoma or parathyroid hyperplasia caused by renal dysfunction may induce adhesion to the surrounding organs, so that they rarely descend, parathyroid adenoma or primary hyperplasia of the parathyroid may lead the glands to descend caudally because they have no supporting structure except for the feeding vessels. The upper parathyroid glands are commonly located behind the recurrent laryngeal nerves, and sometimes are located between the esophagus and trachea. The lower glands are commonly located on the anterior side of the recurrent laryngeal nerves.

c. Supernumerary parathyroid glands

The usual number of parathyroid glands is four. Some reports have indicated that only three glands could be detected, although it is sometimes difficult to conclude whether this was the true number in that case or represented a failure during the search for the glands. On the other hand, supernumerary glands (five or more glands), are often detected. The clinical significance of this condition is that can be a cause of continuing hyperparathyroidism (2, 4). The most common cause of supernumerary glands is when a part of the parathyroid gland is detached during the process of the embryological development of the parathyroid gland. In approximately two-thirds of the cases, the supernumerary gland is found below the thyroid, in association with the thyrothymic ligament or the thymus, while one-third of these glands are found in the vicinity of the thyroid (2). The separated glands are called "rudimentary glands", which are only minimally (less than 5 mg) separate from the parathyroid gland, or "split glands", which are separated evenly. In general, these supernumerary glands are smaller than the normal glands.

6. The uncommon location in this case

In the present case, the enlarged parathyroid gland was considered to be the right lower gland, although Wang et al reported that the intrathyroidal parathyroid was generally the upper gland (4). They indicated that the primordium of the parathyroid gland in the fourth branchial pouch is trapped between the lateral and the median thyroid prior to their embryological fusion. Indeed, most intrathyroidal parathyroid glands are located in the middle or the lower third of the thyroid. In the 1980s, there was a disagreement about the embryonic origin of intrathyroidal parathyroid adenoma. However, a contrary opinion, considering that the intrathyroidal parathyroid adenomas were derived from the lower gland, was also estimated by some researchers. Recently, some reports have shown that the intrathyroidal parathyroid gland can correspond to upper, lower or supernumerary glands (7).

In our case, the upper gland was normal, which suggests that the intrathyroidal parathyroid can be considered to be the lower gland. Our hypothesis is that the lower parathyroid descended incompletely in the sinus of the middle of the thyroid lobe, and the crease had sealed over time. However, regardless of whether an intrathyroidal parathyroid gland is the upper, the lower or a supernumerary gland, we consider that the parathyroid descent to the crease or the sinus of the thyroid and develop toward the inside of the thyroid parenchyma during the embryonic process.

7. Discussion

The incidence of the intrathyroidal parathyroid glands is about 1-4%, and adenoma is the most common cause of persistent hyperparathyroidism among hyperparathyroid patients (5, 7). Moreover, most of the affected glands are located in the right lobe. The choice of treatment for complete resection of intrathyroidal parathyroid adenoma is hemithyroidectomy, instead of parathyroidectomy, because it decreases the incidence of the rupture of the capsule of the parathyroid gland, which could result in a local recurrence.

Despite their wide distribution, the parathyroid glands fall into a definite pattern. Preoperative findings of ultrasound and scinitigram studies may be helpful for identifying localized lesions of intrathyroidal parathyroid adenoma, as well as for intraoperative assessment, which can facilitate the selection of appropriate treatment.

8. Acknowledgements

Written patient's informed consent was obtained for publication of this report.

9. Abbreviations

Primary hyperparathyroidism; PHPT, intact parathyroid hormone; iPTH

10. References

Suliburk JW, Perrier ND: Primary hyperparathyroidism. Oncologist. 12:644-53, 2007

Uludag M, Isgor A, Yetkin G, Atay M, Kebudi A, Akgun I: Supernumerary ectopic parathyroid glands. Persistent hyperparathyroidism due to mediastinal parathyroid adenoma localized by preoperative single photon emission computed tomography and intraoperative gamma probe application. Hormones. 8:144-149, 2009

Yuko Tanaka: Primary hyperparathyroidism with breast carcinoma. Breast Cancer. 17:265-268, 2010

Wang CA: The anatomic basis of parathyroid surgery. Ann Surg. 183: 271-275, 1976

Temmim L, Sinowatz F, Hussein WI, Al-Sanea O, El-Khodary H: Intrathyroidal parathyroid carcinoma: a case report with clinical and histological findings. Diagn Pathol. 25;3:46, 2008

Akerström G, Malmaeus J, Bergström R: Surgical anatomy of human parathyroid glands. Surgery. 95: 14-21, 1984.

Ros S, Sitges-Serra A, Pereira JA, Jimeno J, Prieto R, Sancho JJ, Pérez-Ruiz L: Intrathyroid parathyroid adenomas: right and lower. Cir ESP 84:196-200, 2008

3

Minimally Invasive Parathyroidectomy for Primary Hyperparathyroidism – Current Views, Issues and Controversies

Ian Yu-Hong Wong and Brian Hung-Hin Lang
Department of Surgery, University of Hong Kong
Queen Mary Hospital, Hong Kong SAR
China

1. Introduction

Although primary hyperparathyroidism (pHPT) remains a relatively uncommon endocrine disease in Asian countries with an incidence ranging from 17 to 33 / 100,000 cases per year, it has been increasing over the last decade. (Bilezikian et al. 2000; Lo et al. 2004; Chen et al., 2010) In contrast, in the Western world, pHPT is a relatively more common disease with an estimated incidence of 42 to 190/100,000 cases per year. Surgical treatment or parathyroidectomy remains the only curative therapy for patients with pHPT. The goal of surgery is to normalize postoperative calcium levels by excising all hyperfunctioning parathyroid tissue. Traditionally, this has been achieved by way of bilateral neck exploration (BNE) which involves examination of all four parathyroid glands and excision of any enlarged glands. However, with improvement in preoperative localization techniques and the commercial availability of quick intraoperative parathyroid hormone assay (IOPTH), an increasing number of endocrine surgeons are now performing minimally invasive parathyroidectomy (MIP). In experienced hands, many studies have found that MIP is not only a less invasive procedure associated with shorter hospital stay and less pain but also can achieve similar long-term cure rate of up to 95-98% as BNE which many would still regard it as the gold standard procedure. With this in mind, the purpose of this review is to look at the current views, issues and controversies associated with the use of preoperative localization studies, IOPTH and various surgical techniques of MIP by a comprehensive MEDLINE search using several specific keywords. These keywords include "minimally invasive parathyroidectomy", "focused parathyroidectomy", "intraoperative parathyroid hormone" and "parathyroid adenoma". Since the success of MIP depends partly on the accuracy of preoperative localization studies and IOPTH, it is imperative to assess them in an evidence-based method. The review would look specifically on the use of 99mTc Sestamibi (MIBI) and high-resolution ultrasound (USG) as both modalities are the most commonly employed and accurate imaging before MIP. The review would also look at the issues when there are concordant and discordant results between the MIBI and USG as well as examine the role of surgeon-performed USG (SPUS) in pHPT. Regarding the IOPTH, it remains controversial whether it should be routinely used in all cases of pHPT as some still question the cost-benefit and the "added value" of this particular operative adjunct.

Furthermore, there are still many unresolved issues regarding the most appropriate choice for IOPTH measurements and what criteria for defining biochemical cure. However, it is certain that the recent findings in IOPTH dynamics during MIP have helped us in better understanding of the disease itself. The previous concept of histology and gland size has now been challenged and is gradually being replaced by the concept of biochemical cure based on changes in IOPTH dynamics. Last and not the least, the review will look at various MIP techniques and evaluate which is most commonly used and performed and the reasons behind this.

2. Surgical indications and guidelines

The famous mneumonic "stones, bones, abdominal groans and psychiatric moans" concludes the symptoms of hyperparathyroidism or more specifically hypercalcemia. All patients suffering from the classical symptoms and signs of pHPT should undergo surgical treatment, as it is the only way for cure. On the other hand, the National Institute of Health (NIH) guidelines, as concluded at the third Workshop on the Management of asymptomatic pHPT, had a clear direction for the asymptomatic group of patients to choose between surgery and consideration of medical monitoring. In treating the asymptomatic patients, we are aiming at reversing the decreased bone density, reducing the risk of fractures, reducing frequency of kidney stones and improving the neuro-cognitive elements. The consensus also stressed on the identification of Vitamin D deficiency, as it often complicates the diagnosis of pHPT. Therefore the optimal reference range of PTH assay should be based on adequate Vitamin D repletion, as physiologically, PTH and Vitamin D are closely inter-related.

2.1 Surgical indications for "asymptomatic" patients

According to the NIH guidelines, "asymptomatic" patients with the following features should undergo surgery:

1. Hypercalcemia with serum calcium >1mg/dl above the upper limits of normal;
2. Peri or post menopausal women, and men age >50 with a bone density T-score of -2.5 or less at the lumbar spine, femoral neck, total hip or 33% radius; Premenopausal women and in men younger age <50 with the bone density Z-score of -2.5 or less; Any patient with the presence of a fragility fracture.
3. Age less than 50

Table 1 summarized the changes in surgery criteria in the last decade. In the 2008 consensus, hypercalciuria was taken out from the guidelines because it is not a specific risk factor for kidney stones in primary hyperparathyroidism. However, it remains an important part of the initial workup to rule out familial hypocalciuric hypercalcemia. There were also questions over the accuracy of glomerular filtration rate (GFR) estimation by creatinine clearance and whether a numeral cut-point was better than an age invariant standard. The new consensus was made, based on the fact that a GFR of less than 60ml/min represented renal insufficiency to the extent that would cause parathyroid hormone elevation. The criteria "fracture fragility" was added to the newest guidelines because apart from bone mineral density, primary hyperparathyroidism would also affect the bone size and structure which in turn influence the fracture proclivity. Patients with age less than 50 were included as part of the targeted group as these patients would have greater risk of complications over time.

Measurement	1990	2002	2008
Serum calcium (>upper limit of normal)	1-1.6 mg/dl	1.0 mg/dl	1.0 mg/dl
24 hour urine for calcium	>400mg/d	>400mg/d	Not indicated
Creatinine clearance (Calculated)	Reduced by 30%	Reduced by 30%	Reduced to <60ml/min
Bone Mineral Density	Z-score <-2.0 in forearm	T-score <-2.5 at any site	T-score <-2.5 at any site and/or previous fracture fragility
Age (yr)	<50	<50	<50

Table 1. Comparison of new and old guidelines for parathyroid surgery in asymptomatic primary hyperparathyroidism

However, guidelines for normocalcaemic hyperparathyroidism were yet to be established with more evidence coming up. Parathyroid surgery should be performed only by highly experienced surgeon, or otherwise failure and complication will be unacceptably high and not cost effective. (Bilezikian et al., 2009)

2.2 Are patients with pHPT truly asymptomatic?

There is increasing evidence that patients with pHPT are not truly asymptomatic and if this proves to be true than all patients with pHPT would theoretically benefit from surgery. As a surgeon, it is not uncommon to see that patients with mild evidence of depression and anxiety at preoperative visits often improve after a successful parathyroidectomy. One of the explanations for this is that it is believed that there is a strong link between serum calcium levels and cognitive function. (Roman et al., 2011) In a general population cohort study of more than 4000 individuals, Schram et al. found that high serum calcium levels were associated with faster decline in cognitive function, especially for people older than 75 years. This finding persisted even if people with abnormally high serum calcium levels were excluded.(Schram et al, 2007) Weber et al. evaluated 66 patients who underwent parathyroidectomy for pHPT pre-and postoperatively with 2 validated psychometric instruments and a health-related quality of life health survey (SF-12). They found that patients had significantly more depression and anxiety preoperatively than at 1 year postoperatively, whereas their physical functioning did not change. In this study, preoperative neuropsychological symptoms were related to the serum calcium levels.(Weber et al, 2007) Roman et al. studied 55 patients undergoing either parathyroidectomy for pHPT or thyroid resection for benign thyroid disease as controls and compared their neurocognitive test scores and psychological symptoms before and after surgery. They found that patients with pHPT reported more symptoms of depression and showed greater delays in spatial learning preoperatively than patients with thyroidectomy, but they improved significantly 1 month after surgery at a level equivalent to the controls. Interestingly, patients with greater change in PTH levels were more likely to improve in their learning efficiency after parathyroidectomy. (Roman et al., 2005) The same group also recently assessed the timing and magnitude of psychological and neurocognitive changes before and after parathyroidectomy and found significant improvements in psychological and neurocognitive measures at all postoperative visits. The most pronounced improvements were noted in depressive and anxiety symptoms, and visuospatial and verbal memory. Examination of change scores revealed that postoperative reduction in PTH was associated with a decrease in state anxiety, which was also associated with improvement in visuospatial working memory.(Roman et al., 2011)

3. Preoperative parathyroid localization

Accurate preoperative localization plays a pivotal role in the success of MIP. Numerous imaging techniques such as technetium Tc99m sestamibi imaging (MIBI), high-resolution ultrasound (USG), magnetic resonance imaging (MRI), and computed tomography (CT) have been used to guide the surgeon and to assist with the preoperative planning. Among these imaging studies, MIBI and / or USG have been the two most commonly used preoperative imaging modalities because they are both readily available and relatively inexpensive. MRI and CT have also been advocated as second-line localization modalities as they do not appear to have better accuracy than MIBI or USG but they can localize inferiorly located or deeply seated parathyroid glands (e.g. mediastinal adenoma). When comparing the accuracy in detecting abnormal parathyroid glands between MIBI and USG, some have found that MIBI is more accurate than USG while other studies have found the opposite or similar accuracies. (Cheung et al., 2011) In our experience, MIBI has a higher overall sensitivity, accuracy and positive predicted value (PPV) in detecting abnormal parathyroid glands than USG (85%, 97% vs 94% vs. 57% vs 89%, 56%, respectively). (Lo et al., 2007) In fact, at our institution, we would rely more on the findings of the MIBI than USG. However, since USG could provide additional localization information in approximately 10-15% of patients with negative or equivocal MIBI, we have not abandoned the use of USG as a preoperative localizing tool.(Lo et al., 2007) In our clinical practice, all biochemically-confirmed pHPT patients would undergo MIBI and if the MIBI is negative or equivocal, an additional USG by our radiologists would be performed. However, we would still perform an intraoperative USG by ourselves just before the skin incision to guide the placement of the small skin incision. Our experiences with MIBI and USG have been consistent with those of other institutions. Quiros et al. reported their experience on 71 patients with pHPT who underwent both preoperative MIBI-SPECT and USG and found that if the MIBI was either negative or "ambiguous", preoperative USG could localize an additional 14% of enlarged parathyroid glands and so further facilitate MIP in these patients.(Quiros et al., 2004) Similarly, Adler et al. recently evaluated the added benefit of USG to MIBI in pHPT and reported that USG led to additional localization information in 14% of patients, although this benefit was less in patients with a clearly positive 1-gland MIBI scan. (Adler et al, 2011) Apart from MIBI and USG, 4D-CT has been shown to be a promising adjunct to other imaging studies. 4D-CT could provide exquisitely detailed, multiplanar images that accentuate the differences in the perfusion characteristics of hyperfunctioning parathyroid glands (i.e. rapid uptake and washout), compared with normal parathyroid glands and other structures of the neck.(Starker et al., 2011) In contrast to other axial imaging studies such as CT or MRI, the 4D-CT images could provide both anatomical information (which is vital for the surgeon) and functional information based on changes in perfusion in a single study. Starker et al. compared 4D-CT with MIBI and USG for parathyroid localization and found that 4D-CT had improved sensitivity (85.7%) over MIBI (40.4%) and USG (48.0%) in parathyroid localization. (Starker et al., 2011) Similarly, Cheung et al. recently reported the results of a meta-analysis of preoperative localization techniques which included MIBI, USG and 4D-CT in patients with pHPT. They found a total of 43 studies which met their inclusion criteria and of these, 19 studies were on USG, 9 studies on MIBI-SPECT and 4 studies on 4D-CT studies. USG had pooled sensitivity and PPV of 76.1% and 93.2%, respectively whereas MIBI-SPECT had a pooled sensitivity and PPV of 78.9% and 90.7%, respectively. 4D-CT had the highest sensitivity and PPV of 89.4% and 93.5%, respectively. Therefore, the authors concluded that MIBI-SPECT and USG had similar localization ability but 4D-CT may have improved accuracy. (Cheung et al., 2011)

3.1 Patients with negative preoperative localization studies

Patients with negative imaging represent an important subset of patients with pHPT because of increased frequency of multiglandular disease (38% vs 15% in patients with positive localization study). (Chan, R. K. et al., 2008) Because of the higher incidence of multiglandular disease, surgery needs to be conducted with a level of suspicion that multiglandular disease exists to ensure that all diseased glands are resected during the operation. In our experience, those with scan-negative and USG-negative results had significantly smaller sized parathyroid adenomas even if they only suffered from single gland disease.(Lo et al., 2007). The incidence of both MIBI- and USG-negative patients ranged between 12 - 18%. (Lo et al., 2007) One study compared the parathyroid histology between those with negative MIBI and with positive MIBI.(Mihai et al., 2006) They found that those with negative MIBI had a higher incidence of chief cells than those with positive MIBI, who had a higher incidence of oxyphilic cells. (Mihai et al., 2006)

4. Surgical management

While surgical intervention remains the only curative therapy for patients with hyperparathyroidism, conventional BNE with resection of enlarged parathyroid gland was the gold standard for treatment of pHPT. With the emerging preoperative and intraoperative localization technique as discussed in previous sections, focused-approach or MIP is coming to the throne.

4.1 Definition of cure

The general accepted definition of cure in publication is to achieve normocalcemia for at least 6 months postoperatively. Operative failure or persistent disease is defined as presence of hypercalcemia within 6 months of parathyroidectomy. Recurrent disease can be defined as recurrence of hypercalcemia after 6 months postoperative.

4.2 Surgical options

4.2.1 Conventional BNE

BNE is the traditional surgical approach for management of pHPT. In general it gives a successful rate of greater than 95% and with complication rate of less than 4%. It involved a classic transverse incision at skin crease of about 5cm. All 4 parathyroid glands were identified and examined. All the morphologically abnormal glands were removed. IOPTH can be used as an adjunct for confirmation of cure. In case the IOPTH was negative, extra dissection may be needed to identify ectopic glands. A delayed second stage operation with relocalization by imaging can be considered if ectopic glands could not be found intraoperatively. (Augustine et al., 2011)

4.2.2 MIP

MIP has now become the standard approach for surgical management of pHPT. It is the approach of choice for patients diagnosed with pHPT caused by a solitary parathyroid adenoma, and it is fast becoming an alternative approach in parathyroid reoperations. It comes in various forms and under various names; these include total endoscopic approach, video-assisted approach, radio-guided approach and mini-incision approach. In principle, however, they are similar, as they involve surgical excision of one single abnormal parathyroid gland (ie, adenoma) without disturbing the other three parathyroid glands. Therefore, a better collective name for them should be the focused approach.

Although the extracervical approaches have been described for both unilateral and BNE, they have not been adopted widely. (Ikeda et al. 2000; Lang 2010) Among the endocrine surgeons, the most popular approach remains the open mini-incision approach with no video assistance. The mini-incision approach in MIP is technically similar to the one in MIT. Essentially a 2 cm incision is made at the medial border of SCM. The site of incision is marked after performing a bedside USG in the operating theater. The incision site is placed close to the localized parathyroid adenoma such that minimal tissue dissection is required. Like the mini-incision approach in MIT, a subplatysmal space is developed, and the plane between SCM and strap is opened up. Once the common carotid artery is identified, it is important to dissect all the way down to the prevertebral fascia medial to the artery such that the thyroid lobe and parathyroid glands can be retracted medially. At this point, the parathyroid adenoma usually is identified and carefully excised in whole.

MIP is an operation associated with low morbidity and high success rates (greater than 95%), but the operating surgeon should be meticulous, familiar with the anatomy, and experienced. Unlike the traditional open method where all four parathyroid glands are identified, MIP requires accurate preoperative localization of the abnormal parathyroid gland before it can be attempted. This is because in MIP, the operating surgeon would not have the benefit of examining the other three parathyroid glands; therefore, there is a possibility of missing underlying multiglandular disease such as double adenomas or four-gland hyperplasia. In the author's center, over 70% of patients with newly diagnosed pHPT will be eligible for MIP because of a positive preoperative localization by MIBI or USG. (Lo et al. 2007) To further improve the surgical success of MIP and to minimize the possibility of persistent or recurrent HPT after MIP, some have advocated the routine use of various surgical adjuncts such as radioguided probes or a quick IOPTH at the time of operation, but to date, their routine use remains questionable because of the marginal benefit and the high cost-to-benefit ratio. Nevertheless, MIP with or without the use of adjuncts, when performed in experienced hands has an equivalent success rate of greater than 95%, as the conventional four-gland exploration, and has all the benefits one expects from minimally invasive surgery.

Similar to other minimally invasive procedures, MIP, when compared to conventional BNE, has obvious advantages as it decreases surgical morbidity in terms of cosmesis, pain, risk of recurrent laryngeal nerve injury, postoperative hypocalcaemia, etc. It can also reduce the cost, as well as the operative time and hospital stay. It is, in fact, currently an ambulatory surgery in many centres. Base on the fact that majority ~90% of patients with pHPT are having single hyperfunctioning adenoma, preoperative localization imaging can often narrow down the pathology to the specific quadrant. A smaller, e.g. 2cm, incision is made over the suspected location of the adenoma. The authors adopted the lateral approach with dissection through the plane between the sternocleidomastoid muscle and the strap muscles. Dissection continued medial to the carotid artery to identify the prelocalised enlarged adenoma behind the thyroid gland. IOPTH can give extra confidence to the surgeon and to confirm cure of the disease. As we shall see later, there are increasing evidence that perhaps IOPTH may not be necessary, base on the fact that there is a high specificity of preoperative localization technique, especially in concordant MIBI and SUS. Udelsman et al. published data demonstrating the superior cure rate of MIP of 99.4% as compared to standard BNE of 97.1%.(Udelsman et al 2011). Suliburk et al also published the successful rate of MIP was as high as 98% even without IOPTH , depending on case selection.[6] The article also suggested that occult double adenoma was the major reason for failure. Among the 70% of the patients with double adenoma, the IOPTH has actually dropped by more than 50% after the first adenoma was removed. It is suggestive that the second adenoma remained dormant, or its function is suppressed until after the first adenoma is excised. Repeated MIBI scan after first operation can usually localize the second adenoma. On the other hand, in cases with hyperplasia or multiglandular disease (false positive MIBI), IOPTH may be useful. (Suliburk et al., 2011) [table 1] showed the published article on the outcome of MIP (Starker et al., 2011).

4.2.3 Endoscopic/video-assisted parathyroidectomy

Similar to MIP, endoscopic or video-assisted parathyroidectomy required accurate preoperative localization. Endoscopic instruments often provide better visualization of anatomic structures because of better lighting and magnification. An extra advantage of endoscope is that it can also facilitate mediastinal exploration from a transcervical approach.

5. IOPTH

Despite the fact that IOPTH has been commercially available for over 20 years, the issue of whether to routinely use it in MIP still remains unresolved. The arguments against its use mainly relates to the extra cost of the assay, the extra time required for the result to come back (i.e. extra theatre time), the inability in detecting multiglandular disease on some occasions and the limited added value in some select cases.(Stalberg et al., 2006; Suliburk, J. W. et al., 2011) Some groups without using IOPTH achieved similar cure rate as those with IOPTH. (Cho et al., 2011; Suliburk et al., 2011) As a result, some groups have advocated the use of IOPTH more selectively or in some situations such as in cases of discordant or equivocal localization studies. Kebebew et al. formulated a scoring system for this and suggested that patients with a score of 3 or more do not require IOPTH whereas a score of less than 3 would benefit from IOPTH. (Kebebew et al., 2006) Although these arguments may be true, most surgeons including us still prefer using IOPTH routinely in MIP. Some would argue that it is the "feel-good" factor which is important when performing this sort of a limited, focused approach parathyroidectomy because the surgeon do not have the benefit of looking at the other parathyroid glands and furthermore, the surgeon would be able to tell the patients and their relatives confidently that the IOPTH did drop after excision of the parathyroid gland.

First Author, Journal, year	Study design	Patient No.	Preoperative localization method	Success rate	Intraoperative Adjuncts	Criteria
Untch et al; J Am Coll Surg; Apr 2011	Retrospective, 2001-2010	516	MIBI +/- USG	99.00%	IOPTH	50% reduction + normal
Suliburk et al; ANZ J Surg; Feb 2010	Retrospective, 1998-2008	1020	MIBI + USG	97.80%	No IOPTH	n/a
Hwang et al; Ann Surg; Jun 2010	Prospective, 2006-2009	280	MIBI-SPECT + USG	97.90%	IOPTH in USG +ve/MIBI -ve	Miami criterion (50% reduction)
Lew et al; Surgery; Dec 2009	Retrospective, 1993-1998	173	MIBI	98.00%	IOPTH +/- BIJVS	Miami criterion (50% reduction)
Lew et al; Arch Surg; Jul 2009	Retrospective, 1993-2009	845	MIBI +/- USG	97.10%	IOPTH	Miami criterion (50% reduction)
Gill et al; Otolaryngol Head Neck Surg; Feb 2011	Retrospective 2005-2009	83	MIBI	97.00%	IOPTH	Miami criterion (50% reduction)
Udelsman et al; Ann Surg; Mar 2011	Retrospective 1998-2009	1037	MIBI / USG	99.40%	IOPTH	Miami criterion (50% reduction)
Quillo et al; Am Surg; Apr 2011	Retrospective, 1999-2007	198	MIBI	100% (MIBI neg excluded)	Radioguided	Norman 20% rule
Adil et al; Otolaryngol Head Neck Surg; Mar 2009	Retrospective, 1997-2007	368	MIBI	100% (MIBI neg excluded)	Radioguided	Norman 20% rule
Fouquet et al; Langenbecks Arch Surg; Aug 2010	Retrospective 2001-2008	387	MIBI + USG	98.00%	Total endoscopic lateral parathyroidectomy, IOPTH	Miami criterion (50% reduction)
Politz et al; Endocr Pract; Nov 2006	Retrospective, 2001-2004	118	MIBI	98% (MIBI neg excluded)	Radioguided	n/a
Pang et al; Br J Surg; Mar 2007	Retrospective, 2000-2005	500	MIBI +/- USG	97.40%	No IOPTH	n/a
Mihai et al; Br J Surg; Jan 2007	Retrospective, 2001-2006	298 (150 MIP, 148 BNE)	MIBI + USG	97.30%	No IOPTH	n/a
Cohen et al; Surgery; Oct 2005	Retrospective 1999-2004	139	MIBI-SPECT +/- USG	98.60%	IOPTH	Miami criterion (50% reduction)

Table 2. Summary of recent studies on MIP, respective preoperative localization and intraoperative adjunts.

Nevertheless, the basis for using IOPTH in MIP is that after the removal of the hyperfunctioning or hypersecreting parathyroid adenoma or tissue, the serum PTH would drop and return to its normal range after a certain length of time provided that the remaining unexcised parathyroid glands are normal or not hyperfunctioning. Since the half-life of PTH is only 2-3 minutes in the presence of normal renal function, the recommendation is that one would anticipate a 50% drop from the pre-excision IOPTH level in 10 minutes after excision of the abnormal parathyroid gland. The earliest method for monitoring IOPTH was described by Irvin et al. in 1991 and the recommendation for a 50% decline from preexcision IOPTH level was established in 1993. (Irvin et al., 1991, 1993) This is now known as the "Miami criterion". In this criterion, a successful parathyroid operation is defined as a 50% or more decline from the highest preincision or preexcision IOPTH obtained 10 minutes after excision of the hyperfunctioning parathyroid gland. Therefore, as a surgeon who is using IOPTH, we have shifted the operation end-point from the conventional concept of "abnormal" parathyroid glands based on size and histology in the era of BNE exploration to the current concept of "hyperfunctioning" parathyroid glands with MIP and IOPTH monitoring. However, this shifting in concept still remains somewhat controversial. For example, we recently analyzed 161 consecutive patients who underwent parathyroidectomy (with the majority being MIP) for pHPT at our institution and found that approximately 40% of patients remained to have elevated PTH despite all had normocalcemia (i.e. eucalcemic PTH elevation) at 6-month and had > 50% decline in IOPTH at the time of operation.(Lang et al, 2011) This finding appeared to be consistent to other studies.(Oltmann et al., 2011)) Siperstein et al. showed that preoperative localizing studies and IOPTH failed to identify multiglandular disease in at least 16% of pHPT patients if routine BNE was employed in all patients.(Siperstein et al., 2008) This issue certainly raises concerns on whether by performing MIP and following the IOPTH criterion may lead to higher recurrences in the future. However, in many of the large (>1000 cases) series of image-guided MIP with IOPTH, it is reassuring to find that the long-term cure rate does not appear to be inferior to conventional BNE.(Udelsman et al 2011; Suliburk, J. W. et al, 2011)

The other issue relates to which is the best criterion for IOPTH in terms of highest sensitivity, and accuracy. There have been several studies comparing strategies for IOPTH testing. (Chiu et al., 2006; Carneiro et al., 2003; Barczynski et al., 2009) Barczynski et al. studied 260 patients with presumed solitary parathyroid adenomas based on concordant localization studies. The Miami criterion had the highest accuracy (97%) compared to the Halle (PTH level low normal at 15 minutes), Rome (>50% decline to normal at 20 minutes and / or < 7.5ng/L lower than the 10-minute value), and Vienna (≥50% decline at 10-minutes) criteria. However, in this series, only 3.5% of patients had multiglandular disease and that is comparably low when it is believed that in the era of MIP, the incidence of multiglandular disease would be in the region of 10%. Since multiglandular disease remains one of the biggest downfalls or weaknesses of IOPTH, some groups have advocated to use a more stringent criterion. The Mayo clinic recently reported their experience of 1882 patients. In their series, the incidence of multiglandular disease was 22.0% and they defined a successful exploration as 1 50% or more decline in IOPTH level from baseline and a normal or near-normal IOPTH level at 10 minutes postexcision. They compared this criterion (or the Mayo criterion) with the Miami criterion and found that the Miami criterion would have missed 22.4% of patients with multiglandular disease. They concluded that relying on a 50%

decrease alone potentially increases the rate of operative failure in patients with multiglandular disease.(Richards et al., 2011) Therefore, it would appear that which is the best IOPTH criterion or strategy depends on the incidence of multiglandular disease at your own institution. In our experience, we believe the Miami criterion is the most convenient crierion, given the fact that we encounter very few multiglandular disease in our locality.(Lang et al, 2010, 2011)

6. References

Adil, E., Adil, T., Fedok, F. et al (2009). Minimally invasive radioguided parathyroidectomy performed for primary hyperparathyroidism. *Otolaryngology - Head and Neck Surgery,* Vol 141, (March 2009), pp.34-38.

Adler, J.T., Chen, H., Schaefer, S. et al (2011) What is the Added Benefit of Cervical Ultrasound to (99m) Tc-Sestamibi Scanning in Primary Hyperparathyroidism? *Annals of Surgical Oncology*.(2011 Apr 21) [Epub ahead of print]

Alvarado, R., Meyer-Rochow, G., Sywak, M. et al. (2010). Bilateral Inthernal Jugular Venous Sampling for Parathyroid Hormone Determination in Patients with Nonlocalizing Primary Hyperparathyroidism. *World Journal of Surgery,* Vol 34(6), (June 2010), pp.1299-1303.

Augustine, M.M., Bravo, P.E., & Zeiger, M.A. (2011). Surgical Treatment of Primary Hyperparathyroidism. *Endocrine Practise.* Vol 17 (Suppl 1), (March-April 2011), pp 75-82,

Barczynski, M., Konturek, A., Hubalewska-Dydejczyk, A. et al. (2009) Evaluation of Halle, Miami, Rome, and Vienna intraoperative iPTH assay criteria in guiding minimally invasive parathyroidectomy. *Langenbecks Archives of Surgery.* Vol.394(5), (September 2009) pp.843-9.

Bilezikian, J.P., Meng, X., Shi, Y. et al. (2000). Primary hyperparathyroidism in women: a tale of two cities—New York and Beijing. *International Journal of Fertility and Women's Medicine.* Vol.45 (March 2000) pp.158–65.

Bilezikian, J.P., Khan, A.A. & Potts, J.T. Jr (2009). Guidelines for the Management of Asymptomatic Primary Hyperparathyroidism : Summary statement from the Thrid International Workshop. *The Journal of Clinical Endocrinology & Metabolism.* Vol. 94(2), (February 2009), pp.335-9, ISSN 0021-972X

Carneiro, D.M., Solorzano, C.C., Nader, M.C. et al. (2003). Comparison of intraoperative iPTH assay (QPTH) criteria in guiding parathyroidectomy: which criterion is the most accurate? *Surgery.* Vol 134(6), (December 2003), pp.973-9; discussion pp. 979-81

Chan, R.K., Ruan, D.T., Gawande, A.A. et al. (2008) Surgery for Hyperparathyroidism in Image-Negative Patients. *Archives of Surgery.* Vol.143(4), (April 2008), pp.335-337.

Chen, H.H., Chen, Y.W. & Wu, C.J. Primary hyperparathyroidism in Taiwan: clinical features and prevalence in a single-center experience. *Endocrine.* Vol 37(2), (April 2010), pp.373-8.

Cheung, K., Wang, T.S., Farrokhyar, F. et al. (2011) A Meta-analysis of Preoperative Localization Techniques for Patients with Primary Hyperparathyroidism. *Annals of Surgical Oncology*.(2011 June 28). [Epub ahead of print]

Chiu, B., Sturgeon, C., & Angelos, P. (2006) Which intraoperative parathyroid hormone assay criterion best predicts operative success? A study of 352 consecutive patients. *Archives of Surgery*. Vol. 141(5), (May 2006) pp.483-7; discussion pp.487-8

Cho, N.L., Gawande, A.A., Sheu, E.G. et al. (2011) Critical role of identification of the second gland during unilateral parathyroid surgery: a prospective review of 119 patients with concordant localization. *Archives of Surgery*. Vol 146(5), (May 2011) pp.512-6.

Coakley, A.J., Kettle, A.G., Wells, C.P. et al. (1989). 99Tcm sestamibi - a new agent for parathyroid imaging. *Nuclear Medicine Communications*, Vol.10(11), (November 1989), pp.791-4

Cohen, M.S., Finkelstein, S.E., Brunt, L.M. et al. (2005). Outpatient minimally invasive parathyroidectomy using local/regional anesthesia: A safe and effective operative approach for selected patients. *Surgery*, Vol. 138(4), (October 2005), pp.681-7; discussion pp.687-9.

Fouquet, T., Germain, A., Zarnegar, R. et al. (2010). Totally endoscopic lateral parathyroidectomy: prospective evaluation of 200 patients. *Langenbecks Archives of Surgery*, Vol.395(7), (September 2010), pp.935–40.

Fujii, T., Yamaguchi, S., Yajima, R. et al. (2011). Use of Handheld, Semiconductor (Cadmium Zinc Telluride)-Based Gamma Camera in Navigation Surgery for Primary Hyperparathyroidism. *The American Surgeon*, Vol 77(6), (June 2011), pp.690-3.

Gill, M.T., Dean, M., Karr, J. et al (2011). Intraoperative Parathyroid Hormone Assay: A Necessary Tool for Multiglandular Disease. *Otolaryngology – Head and Neck Surgery*, Vol. 144(5), (May 2011) pp.691-7.

Hwang, R.S., Morris, L.F., Ro, K. et al. (2010). A Selective, Bayesian Approach to Intraoperative PTH Monitoring. *Annals of Surgery*, Vol. 251(6), (June 2010) pp1122-6. ISSN 0003-4932/10/25106-1122

Ikeda, Y. & Takami, H. (2000). Endoscopic parathyroidectomy. *Biomedicine & Pharmacotherapy*. Vol 54 Suppl 1, (June 2000) pp.52s-56s.

Irvin, G.L. 3rd, Dembrow, V.D. & Prudhomme, D.L. (1991) Operative monitoring of parathyroid gland hyperfunction. *American Journal of Surgery*. Vol 162(4), (October 1991) pp.299-302

Irvin, G.L. 3rd, Dembrow, V.D. & Prudhomme, D.L. (1993) Clinical usefulness of an intraoperative "quick parathyroid hormone" assay. *Surgery*. Vol 114(6), (December 1993) pp.1019-22; discussion pp.1022-3

Ito, F., Sippel, R., Lederman, J. et al. (2007). The Utility of Intraoperative Bilateral Internal Jugular Venous Sampling With Rapid Parathyroid Hormone Testing. *Annals of Surgery*, Vol. 245(6), (June 2007), pp.959-63.

Kebebew, E., Hwang, J., Reiff, E. et al. (2006). Predictors of single-gland vs multigland parathyroid disease in primary hyperparathyroidism: a simple and accurate scoring model. *Archives of Surgery*. Vol 141(8), (August 2006) pp.777-82; discussion pp.782

Lang, B.H. & Lo, C.Y. (2010) Vitamin D3 deficiency is associated with late-onset hypocalcemia after minimally invasive parathyroidectomy in a vitamin D borderline area. *World Journal of Surgery*. Vol 34(6), (June 2010) pp.1350-5

Lang, B.H. (2010) Minimally invasive thyroidectomy and parathyroidectomy : surgical techniques and pearls. *Advances in Surgery*. Vol.44 (2010), pp.185-98

Lang BH, Wong IY, Wong KP et al. (2012) Eucalcemic parathyroid hormone elevation after parathyroidectomy for primary sporadic hyperparathyroidism: risk factors, trend, and outcome. *Ann Surg Oncol*. Vol.19(2):584-90

Lew, J.I. & Irvin, G.L. 3rd (2009). Focused parathyroidectomy guided by intra-operative parathormone monitoring does not miss multglandular disease in patients with sporadic primary hyperparathyroidism: A 10-year outcome. *Surgery*, Vol. 146(6), (December 2009), pp1021-7.

Lew, J.I., Rivera, M., Irvin, G.L. 3rd et al. (2010). Operative Failure in the Era of Focused Parathyroidectomy - A Contemporary Series of 845 Patients. *Archives of Surgery*, Vol 145(7), (July 2010), pp.628-33.

Lo, C.Y., Lang, B.H., Chan, W.F. et al (2007) A prospective evaluation of preoperative localization by technetium-99m sestamibi scintigraphy and ultrasonography in primary hyperparathyroidism. *American Journal of Surgery*.Vol 193(2), (February 2007) pp.155-9

Lo, C.Y., Chan, W.F., Kung, A.W. et al. (2004). Surgical treatment for primary hyperparathyroidism in Hong Kong: changes in clinical pattern over 3 decades. *Archives of Surgery*. Vol. 139(1), (January 2004), pp.77-82; discussion pp.82

Mihai, R., Gleeson, F., Buley, I.D. et al. (2006) Negative imaging studies for primary hyperparathyroidism are unavoidable: correlation of sestamibi and high-resolution ultrasound scanning with histological analysis in 150 patients. *World Journal of Surgery*. Vol.30(5), (May 2006), pp.697-704.

Mihai, R., Palazzo, F.F., Gleeson, F.V. et al. (2007) Minimally invasive parathyroidectomy without intraoperative parathyroid hormone monitoring in patients with primary hyperparathyroidism. *British Journal of Surgery*, Vol. 94(1), (January 2007) pp. 42-7

Mihai, R., Simon, D. & Hellman, P. (2009). Imaging for primary hyperparathyroidism - an evidence-based analysis. *Langenbecks Archives of Surgery*, Vol 394(5), (September 2009), pp.765-84.

Modarai, B., Sawyer, A., Ellis, H. (2004). The glands of Owen. *Journal of the Royal Society of Medicine*, Vol 97(10), (October 2004), pp.494-5

Murphy, C. & Norman, J. (1999). The 20% rule : a simple, instantaneous radioactivity measurement defines cure and allows elimination of frozen sections and hormone assays during parathyroidectomy. *Surgery*, Vol 126(6), (December 1999), pp.1023-8; discussion pp.1028-9.

Oltmann, S.C., Maalouf, N.M., Holt, S. (2011) Significance of elevated parathyroid hormone after parathyroidectomy for primary hyperparathyroidism. *Endocrine Practice*, Vol 17 Suppl 1 (March–April 2011) pp.57-62

Pang, T., Stalberg, P., Sidhu, S. et al. (2007). Minimally invasive parathyroidectomy using the lateral focused mini-incision technique without intraoperative parathyroid hormone monitoring. *British Journal of Surgery*, Vol. 94(3), (March 2007), pp. 315-9

Politz, D., Livingston, C.D., Victor, B. et al. (2006). Minimally invasive radio-guided parathyroidectomy in 152 consecutive patients with primary hyperparathyroidism. Endocrine Practice, Vol 12(6), (November –December 2006), pp.630-4.

Quillo, A.R., Bumpous, J.M., Goldstein, R.E. et al. (2011). Minimally Invasive Parathyroid Surgery, The Norman 20% Rule: Is It Valid. *The American Surgeon*, Vol 77(4), (April 2011), pp.484-7

Quiros, R.M., Alioto, J., Wilhelm, S.M. et al. (2004) An algorithm to maximize use of minimally invasive parathyroidectomy. *Archives of Surgery*, Vol.139(5), (May 2004), pp.501-6; discussion pp.506-7

Richards, M.L., Thompson, G.B., Farley, D.R. et al. (2011). An Optimal Algorithm for Intraoperative Parathyroid Hormone Monitoring. *Archives of Surgery*, Vol 146(3), (March 2011), pp.280-5.

Roman, S.A., Sosa, J.A., Mayes, L. et al. (2005). Parathyroidectomy improves neurocognitive deficits in patients with primary hyperparathyroidism. *Surgery*. Vol.138(6), (December 2005) pp.1121-8; discussion pp.1128-9.

Roman, S.A., Sosa, J.A., Pietrzak, R.H. et al. (2011). The effects of serum calcium and parathyroid hormone changes on psychological and cognitive function in patients undergoing parathyroidectomy for primary hyperparathyroidism. *Annals of Surgery*, Vol. 253(1) (January 2011), pp.131-7.

Schram, M.T., Trompet, S., Kamper, A.M. et al. (2007). Serum calcium and cognitive function in old age. *The Journal of the American Geriatrics Society*. Vol. 55(11), (November 2007), pp.1786-92.

Siperstein, A., Berber, E., Barbosa, G.F. et al. (2008) Predicting the success of limited exploration for primary hyperparathyroidism using ultrasound, sestamibi, and intraoperative parathyroid hormone: analysis of 1158 cases. *Annals of Surgery*. Vol. 248(3), (September 2008) pp420-8.

Stalberg, P., Sidhu, S., Sywak, M. et al. (2006) Intraoperative parathyroid hormone measurement during minimally invasive parathyroidectomy: does it "value-add" to decision-making? *Journal of the American College of Surgeons*.Vol 203(1), (July 2006) pp.1-6. Epub 2006 May 30

Starker, L.F., Fonseca, A.L., Carling, T. et al. (2011). Minimally invasive Parathyroidectomy. *International Journal of Endocrinology*. Vol. 2011:206502, (May 2011) Epub 2011 May 23.

Starker, L.F., Mahajan, A., Björklund, P. et al. (2011) 4D parathyroid CT as the initial localization study for patients with de novo primary hyperparathyroidism. *Annals of Surgical Oncology*. Vol 18(6), (June 2011) pp.1723-8.

Suliburk, J.W., Sywak, M.S., Sidhu, S.B. et al (2011). 1000 minimally invasive parathyroidectomies without intra-operative parathyroid hormone measurement: lessions learned. *ANZ Journal of Surgery*,Vol. 81(5), (May 2011), pp362-5

Udelsman, R., Lin, Z. & Donovan, P. (2011). The Superiority of Minimally Invasive Parathyroidectomy Based on 1650 Consectuive Patients With Primary Hyperparathyroidism. *Annals of Surgery*, Vol. 253(3), (March 2011,) pp.585-91. ISSN 0003-4932/11/25303-0585

Untch, B.R., Adam, M.A., Scheri, R.P. et al. (2011). Surgeon-Performed Ultrasound Is Superior to 99Tc-Sestamibi Scanning to Localize Parathyroid Adenomas in Patients with Primary Hyperparathyroidism : Results in 516 Patients over 10 years. *The*

Journal of American College of Surgeon, Vol. 212(4), (April 2011), pp.522-9 ; discussion pp.529-31.

Weber, T., Keller, M., Hense, I. (2007). Effect of parathyroidectomy on quality of life and neuropsychological symptoms in primary hyperparathyroidism. *World Journal of Surgery*. Vol. 31(6), (June 2007), pp.1202-9.

4

Radio-Guided Surgery and Intraoperative iPTH Determination in the Treatment of Primary Hyperparathyroidism

Paloma García-Talavera and José Ramón García-Talavera
Universidad de Salamanca
Spain

1. Introduction

Different opinions exist regarding surgical techniques in the case of primary hyperparathyroidism (PHPT). Traditionally, all patients who underwent surgery were given a bilateral neck exploration.

Since the main cause of PHPT is solitary adenoma, Tibblin et al. (1982) described the possibility of performing a unilateral neck exploration. Up till that time, the greatest limitation for this technique was the lack of precision in preoperative localization protocols. Nowadays, thanks to ^{99m}Tc-methoxy-isobutyl-isonitrile (MIBI) scintigraphy (Fig 1) and high resolution ultrasonography, unilateral neck exploration is successfully applied. ^{99m}-Tc-MIBI imaging has been widely acknowledged as a basic test for preoperative localization and planning of the operation, being the test of choice in patients with persistent or recurrent PHPT, suspect of ectopic adenomas or in those who have been submitted to thyroidectomy or to other previous neck operations (Papathanassiou et al., 2008).

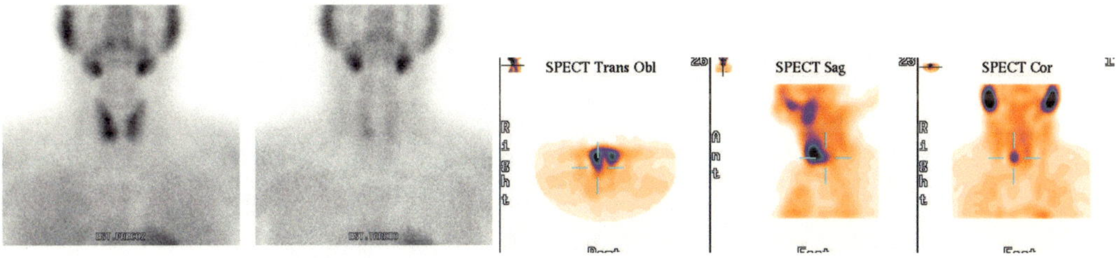

Fig. 1. Double phase ^{99m}Tc-MIBI scintigraphy: Planar images and early SPECT in a patient with a right inferior single adenoma.

Besides, in many occasions, intraoperative intact parathyroid hormone (ioPTHi) detection allows a unilateral neck approach, avoiding extensive surgery and increasing success rates.

Moreover, due to the use of other intraoperative methods, such as the gamma probe, it is possible to perform even more limited surgery (minimally invasive parathyroidectomy -MIP). At some medical centres, the combination of these techniques has allowed to perform outpatient surgery, with a clear benefit from the cost-efficiency point of view, compared to general anaesthesia and much more extensive cervical dissection. Nevertheless, it should be kept in mind that in the case of minimally invasive methods patients must be carefully selected to make sure there is no multiglandular disorder (e.g., MEN or secondary hyperparathyroidism).

Another intraoperative technique which needs further investigation is the use of portable gamma-cameras. As yet few studies with a limited number of patients have been published concerning this new technique.

Consequently, PHPT surgical treatment differs in accordance with the surgeon's preference and the availability of preoperative techniques.

2. Gamma probe

The same year when Norman & Chheda (1997) proposed the use of ^{99m}Tc-MIBI mapping to guide minimally invasive parathyroidectomy, Bonjer et al. (1997) suggested using a probe during a bilateral cervical exploration for intraoperative detection of parathyroid adenomas not visualised preoperatively by scintigraphy.

The technique of intra-operative gamma-detection is based on the differences between the kinetics of MIBI in hyperfunctioning parathyroid tissue and in its surrounding tissue, including thyroid and lymph nodes. MIBI localizes non-specifically in the mitochondria and cytoplasm in response to elevated membrane potentials across the membrane bilayers. It is concentrated in tissues that have increased cell activity or higher numbers of mitochondria.

The method consist in the intraoperative detection of the tissue to be extirpated, which shows uptake as a result of the radiotracer administered to the patient prior to surgery. Localization is carried out with a manual gamma radiation detector which the surgeon introduces into the surgical field (Fig 2). By means of an acoustic signal and a digital counter measuring over-background radioactive emissions (*in vivo* counting), the damaged tissue is localized and subsequently extirpated.

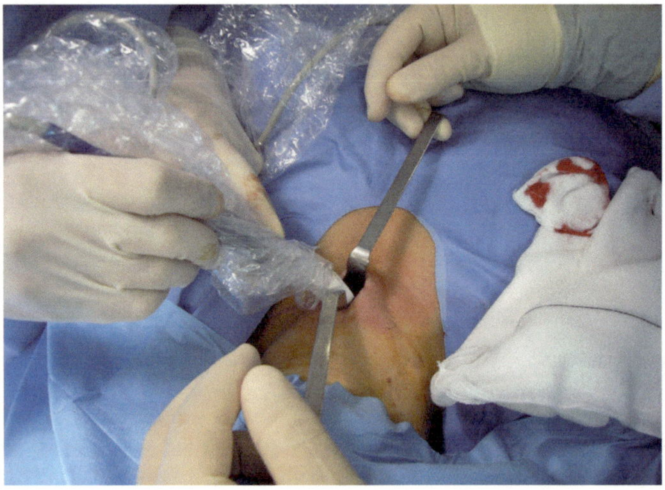

Fig. 2. The surgeon introducing the gamma probe through the incision in a MIP due to a single adenoma.

A further advantage reported is that use of the gamma probe reduces surgery time. In addition, *ex vivo* counting of the extirpated tissue and counting of the empty parathyroid bed, after the excision of the adenoma, serve to assess how successful surgery was.

This technique has been reported a sensitivity between 84.6% and 93% in localizing adenomas, and 63% in the case of disorders compromising multiple glands.

Although this is the traditional way to perform radioguided surgery in hyperparathyroidism, it has been recently reported a case in which authors used a preoperative injection of macroaggregate human albumin (MAA) labeled with ^{99m}Tc into the lesion and ultrasonographic guidance to localize an ectopic parathyroid gland (Aliyev et al., 2010).

2.1 Technique: Doses and time of injection

There is a certain controversy in radioguided surgery with regard to the optimal dose and the optimal time of injection prior to the operative procedure. Norman & Chheda (1997) performed the MIBI scintigraphy on the day of surgery, thus reducing economic cost and radiation doses to the patients. However, in some cases this protocol does not allow planning the type of surgery, while most authors believe that in cases of thyroid pathology a bilateral exploration should be carried out instead of a minimally invasive surgery (Casara et al., 2002). For this reason, in areas of endemic goitre, it is preferable to apply a different-day protocol. Using the latter, Rubello et al. (2006a) propose to carry out a double tracer scintigraphy on the first day and to inject 37 MBq on the day of surgery, 10 to 30 minutes before the minimally invasive parathyroidectomy. In this way, the radiation dose to the surgery team is minimized and false negatives due to parathyroid adenomas with rapid washout are avoided (Rubello et al., 2003).

On the other hand, the time from injection to surgery varies between several minutes (Rubello et al., 2006b) and 3-3.5 h prior to surgery (Dackiw et al., 2000; Mc Greal et al., 2001; Murphy & Norman, 1999), with some authors choosing the proper time depending on when the best ratio is reached between MIBI uptake by the parathyroid tissue and the surrounding tissues (Ugur et al., 2004).

Doses ranging from 37MBq (Rubello et al., 2006b) to 740-925MBq (Goldstein et al., 2003; Mc Greal et al., 2001; Murphy & Norman, 1999) have been reported. In particular, we initially injected 740MBq, 3 h before surgery, but modified our protocol to 370MBq, 10-60 minutes before surgery, in order to reduce radiation doses while keeping the same detection ability.

2.2 Ex vivo and in vivo counting

There are also different approaches regarding the selection of the reference area to measure background: the thyroid gland (Chen et al., 2003, 2005; Takeyama et al., 2004; Ugur et al., 2004, 2006), the lung vertex contralateral to the pathological thyroid gland (Rubello et al., 2003), the right shoulder (Takeyama et al., 2004), the central area of the neck (Goldstein et al., 2003), the lateral region of the incision (Friedman et al., 2007) or the post-exeresis thyroid bed (Mc Greal et al., 2001; Murphy & Norman, 1999; Takeyama et al., 2004; Ugur et al., 2004, 2006).

Takeyama et al. (2004) use the *in vivo* counting as well as the *ex vivo* counting. The *in vivo* counting is used for the localization and removal of the tumor (with the background being obtained as the maximum of two measurements: one on the right shoulder and one on the thyroidal isthmus). The completeness of the excision is confirmed by means of the *ex vivo* counting, which uses the Murphy & Norman procedure (1999) to calculate the corresponding percentage with respect to background.

Ugur et al. (2006) compare the *in vivo* counting of the parathyroid lesion to the thyroidal background of the contralateral side and the *ex vivo* parathyroid counting to the post-exeresis background of the surrounding normal tissues.

Most authors (Chen et al., 2003, 2005; Dackiw et al., 2000; Goldstein et al., 2003; Mc Greal et al., 2001; Murphy & Norman, 1999; Olson et al. 2006; Takeyama et al., 2004), however, use the *ex vivo* counting alone. They confirm a correct exeresis by determining the *ex vivo* counting of the specimens and applying the so-called "rule of 20" (i.e., *ex vivo* counts must exceed background by at least 20%). They generally consider the post-exeresis bed as background. When the suspected adenoma is removed, there is a radioactivity decline there and all quadrants show an equal score count (Norman & Chheda, 1997).

According to Rubello et al. (2003a, 2003b), a value for the index determined by the bed and the apex of the lung contralateral to the pathological parathyroid gland close to unity would suggest the complete excision of the hyperactive parathyroidal tissue. These authors (Rubello et al., 2003a) describe an *ex vivo* index (parathyroid gland/background) higher than 40% in all cases of adenoma and in at least one of the pathological parathyroid gland of a multiglandular disease.

Friedman et al. (2007) consider a background measurement made at the skin of the neck, in the lateral zone of the incision. According to their findings, the *ex vivo* counting of the normal parathyroid glands is significantly lower than that of the pathological glands, for which the percentage over background exceeds 40%.

We use the *in vivo* counting to guide surgeon excision. To do so, we obtain a background measurement after incision by placing the probe over the thyroidal isthmus. Once the incision is made, an operative mapping is taken in the four quadrants for bilateral surgeries or in the region of the suspected adenoma for MIP. The *in vivo* index is defined as the ratio of *in vivo* counting to background (García-Talavera et al., 2010, 2011).

The e*x vivo* counting is also used for differentiating between pathological parathyroid tissue and fat, lymphatic nodes, or thymus (Friedman et al., 2007; Norman & Chheda, 1997). We performed this measuring the parathyroid gland outside the operative field (*ex vivo* counting), and comparing it with the empty bed (*ex vivo* index). As stated below, we use the ioPTHi to confirm the complete exeresis of the pathological parathyroid tissue.

2.2.1 Adenoma *vs* hyperplasia

The traditional procedure to differentiate between adenomas and hyperplasic glands is the histological evaluation by frozen section. However, surgeons do not always provide enough tissue to the pathologist or the tissue sections are not cut appropriately, which results in a substantial false positive and false negative rate (Murphy & Norman, 1999). Furthermore, frozen section analysis is often unreliable in distinguishing hyperfunctioning and normally active parathyroid tissue, as this method only provides a view of a single portion of the gland (Irvin & Bagwell, 1979; Murphy & Norman, 1999), with specimens often interpreted as "non diagnostic parathyroid tissue" (Irvin & Bagwell, 1979). Dewan et al. (2005) report that errors in gross tissue evaluation, by both the surgeon and pathologist, give rise to a 6% operative failure rate.

Because of these drawbacks, the *ex vivo* and the *in vivo* counting have been used by some authors to differentiate between adenomas and hyperplasic glands. According to Murphy & Norman (1999), the *ex vivo* counting in adenomas differs from that in hyperplastic glands: <16% radioactivity over background for non-parathyroidal tissues and normal and hyperplastic parathyroid glands *vs* 59±9% (variation range: 18%-136%) for adenomas. Mc Greal et al. (2001) also found statistically significant differences in the *ex vivo* index between single adenomas and other types of tissues; they concluded that, in patients with a MIBI positive scintigraphy, a 20% counting over background for the excised tissue gives a strong evidence of a single adenoma while the counting for lymph nodes, thyroid tissue and normal or hyperplastic glands would not exceed the said value.

On the contrary, Friedman et al. (2007) argue that the *ex vivo* counting can differentiate between pathological parathyroid glands and other tissues, but it is unable to differentiate between adenomas and hyperplasias, given that, although the counting was statistically higher for adenomas than for hyperplasias, the results overlapped in some cases. This view is supported by Chen et al. (2003), who did not find statistically differences between the *in vivo* counting of adenomas and hyperplasias. On the contrary, Ugur et al. (2006), propose an *in vivo* index cut-off value of 103% to differentiate between adenoma and hyperplasic glands, achieving 82.5% sensitivity and 65% specificity.

In our study (García-Talavera et al., 2011), significant differences were found, on one hand, between the *in vivo* index for adenomas and double adenomas (p=0.009) and, on the other, between adenomas and hyperplasias (p=0.002). However for adenomas and multiglandular disease, there is a region of overlapping values. Using a cut-off value of 1.51, we obtained a 67% sensitivity and 87% specificity. With this cut-off value, we reached a PPV of 95% that would allow, in positive cases, to exclude the existence of a second pathological gland with a high confidence. Rubello et al. (2006b) and EANM parathyroid guidelines (Hindié et al., 2009) reported as well that an *in vivo* index greater than 1.5 strongly suggests the presence of a solitary adenoma.

2.2.2 Glandular size

The glandular size and weight have been described to influence the counting of the abnormal glands. Ugur et al. (2004) described a correlation between the *ex vivo* counting and the size of the gland. Thus, he warns that large hyperplasic glands may behave like a parathyroid adenoma as with regard to their total count.

Friedman et al. (2007) concluded, as well, that the percentage of radioactivity above background is proportional to the mass of the specimen, which has significant implications when decision are being made based on radioactive counts obtained from whole excised parathyroid adenomas *vs* biopsy specimens of hyperplastic or normal glands.

On the contrary, in the experience of Chen et al. (2003), gland weight does not directly correlate with *ex vivo* radionuclide counts. They explained that although very large glands tended indeed to have high *ex vivo* counts, the variation range of *ex vivo* counts for smaller glands was very large.

In our experience, a significant non-linear correlation (Spearman, p=0.005) is found between *in vivo* counting and gland volume (García-Talavera et al., 2011).

2.3 Benefits and failures of the probe

The reported benefits of the probe are manifold. As mentioned above, the probe may be used to differentiate between parathyroid adenoma and hyperplasia as well as between pathological parathyroid glands and other macroscopically similar tissues, as for instance, adipose and lymphoid tissues [Murphy & Norman, 1999].

Besides, as often reported (Berland et al., 2005; Chen et al., 2003; Rubello et al., 2003a; Weigel et al., 2005; García-Talavera et al., 2010), an important contribution of the probe is its usefulness in locating ectopic glands: at deep cervical locations, in the mediastinum or in an intrathyroid location.

In particular the gamma probe is very helpful in patients with persistent or recurrent PHPT (Bonjer et al., 1997), and in patients with previous cervical surgery due to thyroid or parathyroid disease (Dackiw et al., 2000). For these patients, the technique allows the extent of reoperation to be minimized reducing complications (Casara et al., 2002). At this point, it must be stated that in cases of persistent disease the failure of the surgery is usually caused by an ectopic adenoma and the detection of this latter improves with the use of the probe.

Compared to the scintigraphy (Chen et al., 2005; García-Talavera et al., 2010, 2011), the probe eliminates FP scintigraphical results, contributing to minimize the extent of surgical intervention. It also avoids the persistence of the disease detecting FN scintigraphic results, because of small adenomas, but especially due to multiglandular disease. This supports the theory that a radioguided surgery can be performed despite a negative scintigraphy (Mc Greal et al., 2001; Rubello et al. 2006b). Dackiw et al. (2000) described possible causes of these negative results: for instance, a relatively weak labeling of the parathyroid tissue with MIBI, relatively small parathyroid adenomas, or background interferences (mediastinal structures, multinodular thyroid gland). In patients with negative scintigraphic results, the advantages of the intraoperative gamma probe over the preoperative scintigraphy include the ability to move interfering structures (thyroid) out of the way of the probe and the ability to perform *ex vivo* counting. Nevertheless, these authors only recommend using intraoperative probe in carefully selected patients with negative or unequivocally MIBI scintigraphies that are undergoing re-operative procedures. In such patients, Norman & Denham (1998) advocated to suppress thyroid function preoperatively with thyroxine.

As previously mentioned, the probe allows verifying the efficacy and completeness of the parathyroidectomy. In this way, it can minimize the extent of dissection (Chen et al., 2003) and allows to perform a MIP, shortening surgery time and hospital stays (Rubello et al., 2003a) thus decreasing costs (Flynn et al., 2000; Goldstein et al., 2000) and improving the esthetic results without major surgical complications.

There are, however, certain shortcomings to radioguided surgery. The most important is its poor use when there is concomitant thyroid pathology (Bonjer et al., 1997). Some authors discourage its use for such patients, since the existence of thyroid nodules with MIBI uptake largely worsens its performance except in those with ectopic or deep cervical adenomas. To detect nodules with a high uptake (which may lead to false positive scintigraphy and errors in radioguided surgery), it has been proposed to acquire a preoperative double-tracer scintigraphy (Casara et al., 2002). Instead, we perform other imaging techniques (ultrasonography, CT or MRI) in addition to the scintigraphy.

The EANM (Hindié et al., 2009) has recently issued guidelines on the application to parathyroidectomy of the gamma detecting probe, as well as scintigraphy and other imagining localization techniques. They review the main indications for the use of the gamma probe, which, as stated above, do not include patients with concomitant thyroid nodules. However, in our experience (García-Talavera et al., 2010), patients with concomitant thyroid pathology should not be excluded *a priori* from MIP, provided that other adjuvant techniques are used along with the gamma probe. The ioPTHi determination can detect FP and indicates whether surgery can be ended or should be continued or converted into a unilateral or bilateral approach.

Another shortcoming is that the sensitivity of the gamma probe decreases in cases of multiglandular desease (Bonjer et al., 1997; Dackiw et al., 2000). The ioPTHi determination has an important role to avoid the rate of FN, as well (García-Talavera et al., 2011).

Despite the many reports supporting radioguided surgery in patients with PHPT, several authors are not so enthusiastic about this technology. Many of them pointed out the high success rate of parathyroidectomy when performed by experienced surgeons and emphasize that radioguided techniques do not routinely provide any additional information. In a series of 60 patients with PHPT, Inabnet et al. (2002) found that although radioguided surgery was helpful in 40% of cases, it provided confusing or inaccurate information in 48% of cases. Jaskowiak et al. (2002) found radoguided technique only helpful in 22% of patients (out of 57 patients with PHPT). However, these authors admit the benefits of this technique in cases of persistent or recurrent PHPT and in the re-operative neck. They added that the gammaprobe localization proved also useful in some cases of ectopic glands.

In our opinion, although the results may vary depending, among other factors, on the skilfulness of surgeon and probe operator, the gamma probe is a useful tool, especially allowing a MIP or unilateral surgery and localizing adenomas in ectopic locations. This technique, in addition to preoperative localization imaging (double phase scintigraphy), increased the overall success rate from 79% to 94% (Table 1), even in a population with a high prevalence of thyroid pathology (García-Talavera et al., 2010). We use this technique as well in reoperations (previous thyroid or parathyroid surgery) with good results, and in bilateral neck exploration where it shortens surgery time and improves the location of ectopic adenomas.

	Without thyroid pathology	With thyroid pathology	Total
Scintigraphy	85.2%	69.7%	79.3%
Scintigraphy & probe	96.3%	90.9%	94.3%
Scintigraphy & ioPTHi	94.4%	93.9%	94.3%
All techniques	98.2%	97.0%	97.7%

Table 1. Success of the combined use of the techniques regarding to the presence or not of concomitant thyroid pathology.

3. Intra-operative intact PTH (ioPTHi)

In the last few years, ioPTHi determination has been incorporated into hyperparathyroidism surgery, as a means of detecting the decrease of this hormone in plasma following excision of all the diseased parathyroid tissue. Information obtained with pre-operative localization procedures, together with the biological confirmation by ioPTHi that the whole hyperfunctioning parathyroid tissue has dried up, makes a unilateral neck approach possible, in many cases, thereby avoiding extensive surgery and increasing the success rate.

In 1988, Nussbaum et al. described a method for rapid ioPTHi detection, namely, by modifying the non-competitive radioimmunoassay technique (IRMA) employed for serum iPTH quantification. Since then, many authors have successfully used this procedure, which requires a radioactive isotope and takes about 30-35 min (from sample collection till the result is available).

Some years later, we saw the commercialisation of a chemiluminescent immunometric assay (ICMA), which has several advantages over the IRMA. With a reduction in total assay time to 15 minutes and without the need for radioactive isotopes, it is even possible to conduct this test in the operating theatre. This technique, developed and documented by Irvin et al. (1993), is being employed, with good results, in surgical treatment of primary and secondary hyperparathyroidism. In a latter study, Irvin & Deriso (1994) assessed that a reduction of more than 50%, ten minutes after excision, is indicative of total extirpation of the diseased parathyroid tissue and highly suggestive of post-operative eucalcemia. With this procedure, they obtained sensitivity and specificity figures of 95% and 100%, respectively.

3.1 Reference values

Carneiro et al. (2003) compared the so-called Miami criterion (ioPTHi drop ≥ 50%, 10 minutes after gland excision, with respect to the maximum of the pre-incision and the pre-excision level,) to other five published criteria used to predict complete resection. In their study, the Miami criterion showed the highest accuracy. The use of any of the others would minimize the false positive results, but would cause unnecessary neck explorations in searching for multiglandular disease.

Riss et al. (2007) compared the incidence of false positives, using three different criteria, specifically, the "Vienna" criterion (> 50% decline of the pre-incision baseline level, 10 minutes after excision), the "Hale" criterion (decline of the ioPTHi level to ≤ 35 pg/ml, within 15 minutes after excision) and the "Miami" criterion. In 207 patients, the use of the Vienna criteria was shown to produce a lower incidence of false positives, thereby decreasing the risk of multiglandular disease when compared to the other criteria evaluated.

Bergson et al. (2004) took samples before skin incision or induction of anesthesia (baseline 1); pre-excision, after identification but before removal of an abnormal gland (baseline 2); at 5 and 10 minutes after gland excision; and at variable intervals thereafter. In cases of multiglandular disease, samples were generally drawn at 10 minutes intervals after each gland was excised. A decresease in ioPTHi level by 50% from baseline 1 and into the normal range (< 65 pg/ml) was used to indicate successful removal of all abnormal parathyroid tissue.

Nevertheless, Thompson et al. (1999) suggested that a cut-off of 70% would result in the identification of a higher proportion of patients with multiglandular disease. On the other hand, Dackiw et al. (2000) proposed that, when using the ioPTHi determination in patients with MEN1, it is reasonable to apply the same target used by Clary et al. (1997) —an approximately 80% decrease in ioPTHi level— in patients with secondary hyperparathyroidism and parathyroid hyperplasia. Analogously, for Hughes et al. (2011), if a multiglandular disease is detected during the operation, a more stringent criterion for determining adequate resection can improve cure rates. They reported that a decrease of ≥ 75% and into the normal range improves the PPV from 93.2 to 96.6, when compared to the standard criterion of a 50% decrease in the ioPTHi baseline level.

We use the classic criteria of a > 50% decrease of ioPTHi, 10 minutes after gland extirpation, compared to the pre-incision level (baseline). As for persistent hyperfunctioning parathyroid tissue, we take samples 10 minutes after every gland excision.

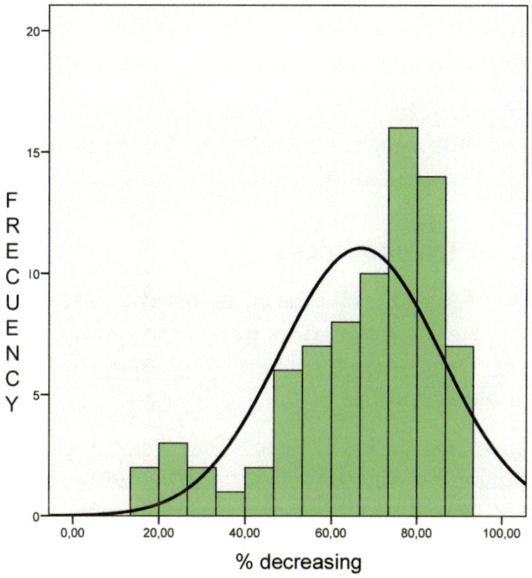

Fig. 3. Distribution of the decresing of the ioPTHi level at 10 minutes in a population of 78 patientes with surgery for PHPT (mean=66.8%; SD=18.8%)
(García-Talavera. Unpublished data).

3.2 Indications

Dackiw et al. (2000) summarize the following main indications of the ioPTHi determination:

1. Predicting clinical cure or indicating the need for bilateral neck exploration and the likehood of multiglandular disease in patients undergoing a unilateral or minimally invasive parathyroidectomy.
2. Predicting the cure in patients undergoing an anatomically directed reoperative parathyroidectomy.
3. Indicating the need for additional resection of hyperplasic parathyroid tissue in patients with secondary hyperparathyroidism and MEN1.

4. Suggesting the potential need for autografting and cryopreservation in patients with final ioPTHi values below the lower limit of detection, particularly in patients undergoing a reoperative parathyroidectomy and in patients undergoing a near-total parathyroid excisions.

In addition, the final ioPTHi level has been described to predict those at risk for recurrence after parathyroidectomy. Heller & Blumberg (2009) reported that those patients with a final level of 40 pg/ml or higher are at risk of having persistent hyperparathyroidism and should be followed-up closely and indefinitely following parathyroidectomy.

The ioPTHi determination has been described, as well, to be useful in detecting false negatives of imaging techniques. Sugino et al. (2010) divided patients who underwent minimally invasive parathyroidectomy into two groups, depending on the determination or not of the ioPTHi. The overall cure rate increased from 93.1%, in the group without ioPTHi determination, to 97.5%, in the group with ioPTHi. These authors concluded that although preoperative localization studies are accurate and essential, ioPTHi monitoring improves the cure rate. The ioPTHi monitoring is a valuable adjunct to achieve adequate intraoperative decision-making, recognizing and resecting additional image-negative hyperfunctioning lesions.

Finally, as mention before, it is a useful tool to detect false positives of the gamma probe in patients with concomitant thyroid pathology (García-Talavera et al., 2010).

3.3 Controversy on the ioPTHi usefulness

At the beginning, the use of the ioPTHi was considered as a tool with a low rate of failures, but in the last few years several investigators have reported an important rate of inadequate drop of ioPTHi levels in the presence of persistent hyperfunctioning parathyroid tissue, especially in cases of double adenomas.

Haciyanli et al. (2003) support that ioPTHi does not reliably predict double adenomas. The same conclusion was made by Gauger et al. (2010), who reviewed 20 cases of double adenomas identified at bilateral neck exploration, measuring ioPTHi although it was not used to guide surgical decision making. They found that in 55% of the cases, using ioPTHi to make a decision on the removal of all abnormal parathyroid tissue would have resulted in failure to detect the second adenoma. Siperstein et al. (2004) also studied ioPTHi in 350 patients who had been underwent bilateral neck exploration after preoperative 99mTc-MIBI scintigraphy and ultrasonography. If a unilateral exploration based on the imaging test had been performed, ioPTHi level would have failed to predict the presence of multiglandular disease in 9% of patients. Multiglandular disease would have been missed in 15% of patients if a MIP had been performed.

However, there are a lot of publications advocating for the use of this technique to improve the success of parathyroidectomy. Furtheremore, ioPTHi determination has been reported as the most accurate predictor of multiglandular disease (Sugg et al., 2004). In a smaller series, Stratmann et al. (2002) found that the ioPTHi measurement accurately predicted the presence of multiglandular disease in 8 out of 8 patients with PHPT suspected of having a solitary adenoma on preoperative MIBI scintigraphy. Kandil et al. (2009) studied 47 patients with double adenomas and concluded that ioPTHi monitoring accurately predicted the success of parathyroidectomy in 98% of patients with double adenomas.

In our experience, as we previously mentioned, the ioPTHi determination is a valuable method to detect FN of the gamma probe due to multiglandular disease. Furthermore, in association with the scintigraphy, it improved the success rate in our study from 79% to 94% (Table 1). Despite this fact, we agree with other authors that the ioPTHi technique is not without errors.

3.4 Causes of failures in the ioPTHi technique

Several factors have been associated to the inadequate drop in ioPTHi levels. Some authors have reported false positive decrease in ioPTHi levels, as Zettinig et al. (2002), who described the case of a recurrence hyperparathyroidism due to the existence of a suppressed double adenoma. The theoretical explanation is that in rare occasions smaller abnormal parathyroid glands can be suppressed and may become hypersecretory if they are left *in situ* after surgical removal of the larger gland. Regarding this matter, Sitges-Serra et al. (2010) reported that two-thirds of the patients with double adenomas showed a false-positive decline of ioPTHi after resection of the first adenoma. This appears to be due to the initial removal of the larger lesion when there are marked differences between the two enlarged glands. They think that extending ioPTHi sampling for 15-20 minutes after excision of the first adenoma (in search of a normalization of PTH levels) would be a good choice. Nevertheless, due to the low prevalence of double adenomas, adopting other criteria to define a biochemical intraoperative cure would lead to make surgery more tedious for more than 95% of patients with single gland disease submitted to limited surgery (it prolongs the operating room waiting time too much and may lead to spurious reconversions into bilateral neck exploration). Gordon et al. (1999) support these results; their group, on the validation of the quick ioPTHi assay, included 14 patients with double adenoma. These authors described that 4 of 14 patients with double adenoma cases showed a greater than 50% decrease in ioPTHi after resection of the first lesion, which was always heavier than the second.

Carneiro et al. (2003) specifically analyzed the false positive results in the decrease of ioPTHi in this series. One of them involved an undiagnosed parathyroid cancer, another was due to a verified technical assay error, and the third case had a very high pre-excision level from an intraoperative rupture of a parathyroid cyst.

Another cause of failure in the ioPTHi determination is the existence of false negative decrease of the ioPTHi. Yang et al. (2001) described a possible cause; they reported a spike in parathyroid hormone level during exploration caused by the mobilization of the adenoma. This spike can be unrecognized if baseline values are measured during the early stages. Due to this fact, they changed their protocol by measuring ioPTHi at the time of neck incision, at the time of complete removal of the adenoma, and 10 minutes after excision.

Some authors (Chen et al., 2005) related elder patients and high levels of creatinine to the lack of decrease of ioPTHi after a successful excision. In these cases, the half-life of iPTH may be greater than the 3 to 4 minutes, valid for the majority of patients.

4. Choice among techniques

There are different views regarding the association of intraoperative tools (frozen section, the gamma probe and the ioPTHi determination) during limited parathyroidectomy.

Some (as Jacobson et al., 2004) believe that selected patients with PHPT due to single-gland disease and unequivocally positive preoperative MIBI scintigraphy can safely and successfully be managed with a focused unilateral cervical exploration without either ioPTHi determination or use of the gamma probe. Smith et al. (2009) think, as well, that ioPTHi determination may be eliminated in MIP surgery in a carefully selected group of patients who have preoperative localizing MIBI scintigraphy with concordant US. In their experience, 2 concordant preoperative localization studies result in a 97% rate of successfully performed MIP *vs* an 80% success rate with one positive study alone. In the other hand, adding an ioPTHi measurement in patients with concordant preoperative studies provided only a minor benefit. If the ioPTHi were eliminated in these patients, it would be possible to reduce the cost associated with laboratory fees, operating room time, and anaesthesia time.

Other authors use the ioPTHi determination with previous preoperative imaging techniques. For instance, Bergson et al. (2004) think that preoperative MIBI scintigraphy and ioPTHi measurement allow a successful MIP, with cure rates comparable to traditional results using bilateral neck exploration. In their experience, the ioPTHi allows an accurate identification of multiglandular disease in 88% of cases.

Sidell et al. (2010) support the use of the ioPTHi and frozen section during parathyroidectomy because they help to maximize patient safety, improve confidence, and minimize operative failure.

There are some investigators who support the use of the gamma probe alone, as Murphy & Norman (1999). They state that, if a tissue is removed from a patient with HPTP who has a positive MIBI scintigraphy and this tissue contains more than 20% of the radioactivity in the operative basin, frozen section analysis do not need to be performed and the intraoparative measurement of parathyroid hormone is unnecessary. According to these authors, the use of the ioPTHi is costly, time consuming, applicable primarily to patients with adenomas, and still with errors. In this group, we could include Goldstein et al. (2003) who reported an excellent cure rate for the radioguided MIP technique with a preoperative positive MIBI scintigraphy without ioPTHi determination. But these authors, consider the association of ioPTHi useful in some occasions, such as complicated reoperative settings or suspicion of multiglandular disease.

There are several authors who trust in the association of techniques to achieve the highest success. Dackiw et al. (2000) would always combine preoperative MIBI imaging with the gamma probe and the ioPTHi determination when performing anatomically directed operations, including minimally invasive operations, to help ensure postoperative resolution of hypercalcemia. They claim that the intraoperative gamma probe localization is particularly useful in assisting in the identification of ectopic parathyroid adenomas, whereas the ioPTHi assists in the identification and management of patients with multiglandular deasease. Ugur et al. (2004) compared the *ex vivo* and *in vivo* counting to frozen section, and their conclusion is that the two former methods are more accurate than the latter. On the other hand, they consider the quick ioPTHi assay very helpful, especially in asymmetric hyperplasia cases, because large hyperplastic glands may produce radioactivity countings as high as adenomas do. Chen et al. (2003) found that radioguided surgery facilitated intraoperative localization (especially of ectopically located glands), allowed to give up intraoperative frozen section analysis, and was equally effective for adenomatous and hyperplastic parathyroid glands.

Nevertheless, they believe that the radioguided techniques complement the ioPTHi assay but cannot replace it. In a later publication, these authors (Chen et al., 2005) compared the use of MIBI scanning, radioguided surgery and ioPTHi determination. ioPTHi reached the highest sensitivity (99%), positive predictive value (99.6%) and accuracy (98%). The gamma probe obtained 93%, 88% and 83%, respectively, whereas the scintigraphy achieved 84%, 81%, and 72%, respectively. In the EANM guidelines (Hindié et al., 2011), it is stated that, due to the good ability of the gamma probe to identify hyperactive parathyroid tissue, the probe can replace frozen section, but in order to confirm the complete parathyroid removal the gamma probe should be used in association with ioPTHi measurements. We support as well the combined use of techniques (scintigraphy, gamma probe and ioPTHi), reaching a success rate of 98% (see Table 1).

5. Portable gamma camera

Another useful tool in minimally invasive surgery which still requires more experience and validation is the portable gamma camera. The first portable gamma camera was patented by Soluri et al. (1997) and validated by Scopinaro et al. (1999) for sentinel lymph node biopsy in breast cancer patients. Nowadays these cameras have become smaller and lighter. They have a high degree of sensitivity and spatial resolution, with values approximated to those of the gamma probe. Moreover, dynamic real-time images can be taken, including lateral images of the neck and mediastinal space.

Fuji et al. (2011) used a handheld semiconductor-based gamma camera. They included eleven patients with PHPT and positive scintigraphy, acquiring images before skin incision, after adenoma localization, after adenoma excision, and *ex vivo* imaging of the specimen. The gamma camera allowed them to intraoperatively identify and remove parathyroid adenomas in all cases.

Ortega et al. (2007) made an intra-operative comparison of the utility of a conventional intra-operative probe and a new-generation portable gamma camera. In addition, they determined ioPTHi so as to verify the total extirpation of parathyroid tissue. Consequently, the portable camera could be used together with the intra-operative probe or perhaps it could replace it, as has been suggested by these authors. In a later study, Cassinello et al. (2009) included 20 patients; in 15 cases, ioPTHi was not used for intraoperatively diagnosis and the miniature gamma camera was the only diagnostic tool employed to perform the operation. All cases were successfully operated by a MIP. They concluded that the portable gamma camera can be used as complementary to the standard tools or even to replace them, at least in selected cases of single adenomas.

A possible benefit of this procedure is the application in patients with a thyroid disorder, as illustrated by Ferrer-Rebolleda et al. (2008). However, cost is its biggest disadvantage. As a result, its use would be only justified in centres with a wide range of applications (sentinel lymph node, ROLL, etc.).

6. Conclusion

Nowadays, thanks to the preoperative MIBI scintigraphy and the availability of intraoperative techniques, such as the gamma probe and the ioPTHi determination, MIP can be performed for the surgical treatment of PHPT. This surgical approach improves the aesthetic results, decreases the morbidity and shortens the surgical time, hospital stay and consequently cost, achieving similar successful rates to the bilateral approach.

The benefits of these two techniques (gamma probe and ioPTHi) in bilateral neck exploration have been documented as well. They shorten surgical time and guarantee the completeness of the exeresis of the pathological glands. The general applications of these techniques are the localization of ectopic adenomas (for the gamma probe) and the detection of multiglandular disease (for the ioPTHi test) which have been reported as the main causes of persistent and recurrent PHPT in the traditional surgery. There is a certain controversy over the protocols used (doses, time from injection to surgery, percentage of decrease in ioPTHi…) and accuracy of these tools depending on the authors. Consequently, PHPT surgical treatment differs in accordance with the surgeon's preference and the availability of preoperative techniques.

A new aiding tool in radioguided surgery is the use of the portable gamma camera, combined or not, to other intraoperative techniques. This new device seems to offer good results but further investigation is needed.

7. References

Aliyev, A.; Kabasakal, L.; Simsek, O.; Paksoy, M.; Halac, M. & Uslu, I. (2010). Ectopic parathyroid adenoma localized with MIBI scintigraphy and excised with guide of macroaggregated human serum albumin injection. *Clinical Nuclear Medicine*, Vol.35, No.3 (March 2010), pp. 151-153, ISSN 0363-9762

Bergson, E.J.; Sznyter, L.A.; Dubner, S.; Palestro, C.J. & Heller, K.S. (2004). Sestamibi scans and intraoperative parathyroid hormone measurement in the treatment of primary hyperparathyroidism, *Archives of Otolaryngology- Head & Neck Surgery*, Vol.130, No.1 (Jan 2004), pp. 87-91, ISSN 0886-4470

Berland, T.; Smith, S.L. & Huguet, K.L. (2005). Occult fifth gland intrathyroid parathyroid adenoma identified by gamma probe. *American Surgery*, Vol.71, No.3 (Mar 2005), pp. 264–266.

Bonjer, H.J.; Bruining, H.A.; Pols, H.A.; de Herder, W.W.; Van Eijck, C.H.J.; Breeman, W.A.P.; et al. (1997). Intraoperative nuclear guidance in benign hyperparathyroidism and parathyroid cancer. *European Journal of Nuclear Medicine*, Vol.24, No.3 (March 1997), pp. 246-251, ISSN 0340-6997

Carneiro, D.M.; Solorzano, C.C.; Nader, M.C.; Ramirez, M. & Irvin, G.L. 3rd (2003). Comparison of intraoperative iPTH assay (QPTH) criteria in guiding parathyroidectomy: which criterion is the most accurate? *Surgery*, Vol.134, No.6 (Dec 2003), pp. 973-979, ISSN 0039-6060

Casara, D.; Rubello, D.; Cauzzo, C. & Pelizzo, M.R. (2002). 99mTc-MIBI radioguided minimally invasive parathyroidectomy: experience with patients with normal thyroids and nodular goiters. *Thyroid*, Vol.12, No.1 (Jan 2002), pp. 53-61, ISSN 1050-7256

Casara, D.; Rubello, D.; Pelizo, M.R. & Shapiro, B. (2001). Clinical role of 99mTcO4/ MIBI scan, ultrasound and intraoperative gamma probe in the performance of unilateral and minimally invasive surgery in primary hyperparathyroidism.

European Journal of Nuclear Medicine, Vol.28, No.9, (Sep 2001), pp. 1351–1359, ISSN 0340-6997

Cassinello, N.; Ortega, J. & Lledo, S. (2009). Intraoperative real-time (99m)Tc-sestamibi scintigraphy with miniature gamma camera allows minimally invasive parathyroidectomy without ioPTHi determination in primary hyperparathyroidism. *Langenbeck´s Archives of Surgery*, Vol.394, No.5 (Sep 2009), pp. 869-874, ISSN 0004-0010

Chen, H.; Mack, E. & Starling, J.R. (2003). Radioguided parathyroidectomy is equally effective for both adenomatous and hyperplasic glands. *Annals of Surgery*, Vol.238, No.3 (Sep 2003), pp. 332-338, ISSN 1528-1140

Chen, H.; Mack, E. & Starling, J.R. (2005). A comprehensive evaluation of perioperative adjunts during minimally invasive parathyroidectomy. Which is most reliable? *Annals of Surgery*, Vol.242, No.3 (Sep 2005), pp. 375-383, ISSN 1528-1140

Clary, B.M.; Garner, S.C.; Leight, G.S.Jr. (1997). Intraoperative parathyroid hormone monitoring during parathyroidectomy for secondary hyperparathyroidism. *Surgery*, Vol.122, No.6 (Dec 1997), pp. 1034-1038, ISSN 0039-6060

Dackiw, A.P.B.; Sussman, J.J.; Fritsche, H.A.; Delpassand, E.S.; Stanford, P.; Hoff, A. et al. (2000). Relative contributions of Tc99m Sestamibi scintighaphy, intraoperative gamma probe detection, and the rapid parathyroid hormone assay to the surgical management of hyperparathyroidism. *Archives of Surgery*, Vol.135, No.5 (May 2000), pp. 550-557, ISSN 0004-0010

Dewan, A.K.; Kapadia, S.B.; Hollenbeak, C.S. & Stack B.C.Jr. (2005). Is routine frozen section necessary for parathyroid surgery? *Otolaryngology-Head and Neck Surgery*, Vol.133, No.6 (Dec 2005), pp. 857-862, ISSN 0194-5998

Ferrer-Rebolleda, J.; Sopena, P.; Estremens, P.; Guallart, F.; Reyes, M.D.; Caballero, E. et al. (2008). Aportación de una minigammacámara portatil en el tratamiento quirúrgico del hiperparatiroidismo primario. *Revista Española de Medicina Nuclear*, Vol.27, No.2, (Mar-Apr. 2008), pp. 124-127, ISSN 0212-6982

Flynn, M.B.; Bumpous, J.M.; Schill, K. & McMasters, K.M. (2000). Minimally invasive radioguided parathyroidectomy. *Journal of the American College Surgery*, Vol.191, No.1 (Jul 2000), pp. 24-31, ISSN 1072-7515

Friedman, M.; Gurpinar, B.; Schalch, P. & Joseph, N.J. (2007). Guidelines for radioguided parathyroid surgery. *Archives of Otolaryngoly- Head & Neck Surgery*, Vol.133, No.12 (Dec 2007), pp. 1235–1239, ISSN 0886-4470

Fujii, T.; Yamaguchi, S,.; Yajima, R.; Tsutsumi, S.; Uchida, N.; Asao, T. et al. (2011). Use of a handheld, semiconductor (cadminum zinc telluride)-based gamma camera in navigation surgery for primary hyperparathyroidism. *American Surgery*, Vol.77, No.6 (Jun 2011), pp. 690-693

García-Talavera, P.; González, C.; García-Talavera, J.R.; Martín, M.E.; Martín, M. & Gómez, A. (2010). Radioguided Surgery of primary hyperparathyroidism in a population with a high prevalence of thyroid pathology. *European Journal of Nuclear Medicine & Molecular Imaging*, Vol.37, No.11 (Nov 2010), pp. 2060-2067, ISSN: 1619-7070

García-Talavera, P.; García-Talavera, J.R.; González, C.; Martín, M.E.; Martín, M. & Gómez, A. (2011). Efficacy of in vivo counting in parathyroid radioguided surgery and usefulness of its association with scintigraphy and intraoperative PTHi. *Nuclear Medicine Communications,* Vol. 32, No. 9 (Sep 2011), pp 847-85, ISSN 0143-3636

Gauger, P.G.; Agarwall, G.; England, B.G.; Delbridge, L.W.; Matz, K.A.; Wilkinson, M.; Robinson, B.G. & Thompson, N.W. (2001). Intraoperative parathyroid hormone measurement fails to detect double parathyroid adenomas: a 2-institution experience. *Surgery,* Vol.130, No.6 (Dec 2001), pp. 1005-1010, ISSN 0039-6060

Goldstein, R.E.; Blevins, L.; Delbeke, D. & Martin, W.H. (2000). Effect of minimally invasive radioguided parathyroidectomy on efficacy, lengh of stay, and cost in the management of primary hyperparathyroidism. *Annals of Surgery,* Vol.231, No.5 (May 2000), pp. 732-742, ISSN 1528-1140

Goldstein, R.E.; Billheimer, D.; Martin, W.H. & Richards, K. (2003). Sestamibi scanning and minimally invasive radioguided parathyroidectomy without intraoperative parathyroid hormone measurement. *Annals of Surgery,* Vol.237, No.5 (May 2003), pp. 722-731, ISSN 1528-1140

Gordon, L.; Snyder, W.H.; Wians, F.; Nwariaku, F. & Kim, L.T. (1999). The validity of quick intraoperative parathyroid hormone assay: an evaluation in seventy-two patients based on gross morphologic criteria. *Surgery,* Vol.126, No.6 (Dec 1999), pp. 1030-1035, ISSN 0039-6060

Haciyanli, M.; Lal, G.; Morita, E.; Duh, Q.Y.; Kebebew, E. & Clark, O.H. (2003). Accuracy of preoperative localization studies and intraoparative parathyroid hormone assay in patients with primary hyperparathyroidism and double adenoma. *Journal of the American College of Surgeons,* Vol.197, No.5 (Nov 2003), pp. 739-746, ISSN 1072-7515

Heller, H.S. & Blumberg, S.N. (2009). Relation of final intraoperative parathyroid hormone level and outcome following parathyroidectomy. *Arch Otolaryngol Head Neck Surg,* Vol.135, No.11 (Nov 2009), pp. 1103-1107, ISSN: 0886-4470

Hindié, E.; Ugur, Ö.; Fuster, D.; O´Doherty, M.; Grassetto, G.; Ureña, P. et al. (2009). 2009 EANM parathyroid guidelines. *European Journal of Nuclear Medicine and Molecular Imaging,* Vol.36, No.7 (Jul 2009), pp. 1201–1216, ISSN 1619-7070

Hughes, D.T.; Miller, B.S.; Doherty, G.M. & Gauger, P.G. (2011). Intraoperative parathyroid hormone monitoring in patients with recognized multiglandular primery hyperparathyroidism. *World Journal of Surgery,* Vol.35, No.2 (Feb 2011), pp. 336-341, ISSN: 0364-2313

Inabnet, W.B. III; Kim, C.K.; Haber, R.S. & Lopchinsky, R.A. (2002). Radioguidence is not necessary during parathyroidectomy. *Archives of Surgery,* Vol.137, No.8 (Aug 2002), pp. 967-960, ISSN: 0004-0010

Irvin, G. & Bagwell, C. (1979). Identification of histologically undetectable parathyroid hyperplasia by flow cytometry. *American Journal of Surgery,* Vol.138, N°4 (Oct 1979), pp. 567-571, ISSN 0002-9610

Irvin, G.L. 3rd; Dembrow, V.D. & Prudhomme, D.L. (1993). Clinical usefulness of an intraoperative "quick parathryroid hormone" assay. *Surgery,* Vol.114, No.6 (Dec 1993), pp. 1019-1022, ISSN: 0039-6060

Irvin, G.L. 3rd & Deriso, G.T. (1994). A new practical intraoperative parathyroid assay. *American Journal of Surgery*, Vol.168, No.5 (Nov 1994), pp 466-468, ISSN: 0002-9610

Jacobson SR, van Heerden JA, Farley DR, Grant CS, Thompson GB, Mullan BP, and Curlee KJ. Focused cervial exploration for primary hyperparathyroidism without intraoparative parathyroid hormone monitoring or use of the gamma probe. *World Journal of Surgery*, Vol.28, No.11 (Nov 2004), pp. 1127-1131, ISSN 0364-2313

Jacobson, S.R.; van Heerden, J.A.; Farley, D.R.; Grant, C.S.; Thompson, G.B.; Mullan, B.P. et al. (2004). Focused cervical exploration for primary hyperparathyroidism without intraoperative parathyroid hormone monitoring or use of the gamma probe. *World Journal of Surgery*, Vol.28, No11 (Nov 2004), pp 1127-1131, ISSN: 0364-2313

Jaskowiak, N.T.; Sugg, S.L.; Helke, J.; Koka, M.R. & Kaplan, E.L. (2002). Pitfalls of intraoperative qick parathyroid hormone monitoring and gamma probe localization in surgery for primary hyperparathyroidism. *Archives of Surgery*, Vol.137, No.6 (Jun 2002), pp. 659-668, ISSN: 0004-0010

Kandil, E.; Alabbass, H.H.; Bansal, A.; Islam, T.; Tufaro, A.P. & Tufano, R.P. (2009). Intraoperative Parathyroid hormone assay in patients with primary hyperparathyroidism and double adenoma. *Archives of Otolaryngology- Head & Neck Surgery*, Vol.135, Nº12 (Dec 2009) , pp. 1206-1208, ISSN 0886-4470

McGreal, G.; Winter, D.C.; Sookhai, S.; Evoy, D.; Ryan, M.; O'Sullivan, G.C. et al. (2001). Minimally invasive, radioguided surgery for primary hyperparathyroidism, *Annals of Surgical Oncology*, Vol.8, No.10 (Dec 2001), pp. 856–860, ISSN 1068-9265

Murphy, C. & Norman, J. (1999). The 20% rule: a simple, instantaneous radioactivity measurement defines cure and allows elimination of frozen sections and hormone assays during parathyroidectomy. *Surgery*, Vol.126, No.6 (Dec 1999), pp. 1023–1029, ISSN: 0039-6060

Norman, J. & Chheda, H. (1997). Minimally invasive parathyroidectomy facilitated by intraoperative nuclear mapping. *Surgery*, Vol.122, No.6 (Dec 1997), pp. 998-1004, ISSN: 0039-6060

Norman, J. & Denhan, D. (1998). Minimally invasive radioguided parathyroidectomy in the reoperative neck. *Surgery*, Vol.124, No.6 (Dec 1998), pp 1088-1092, ISSN: 0039-6060

Nussbaum, S.R.; Thompson, A.R.; Hutcheson, K.A.; Gaz, R.D. & Wang, C.A. (1988). Intraoperative measurement of parathyroid hormone in the surgical management of hyperparathyroidism. *Surgery*, Vol.104, No.6 (Dec 1988), pp. 1121-1127, ISSN: 0039-6060

Olson, J.; Repplinger, D.; Bianco, J. & Chen, H. (2006). Ex vivo radioactive counts and decay rates of tisues resected during radioguided parathyroidectomy. *Journal of Surgery Research*, Vol.136, No.2 (Dec 2006), pp. 187-191, ISSN: 0022-4804

Ortega, J.; Ferrer-Rebolleda, J.; Cassinello, N.; Lledo, S. (2007). Potential role of a new hand-held miniature gamma camera in performing minimally invasive parathyroidectomy. *European Journal of Nuclear Medicine and Molecular Imaging*, Vol.34, No.2 (Feb 2007), pp 162-164. ISSN 1619-7070

Papathanassiou, D.; Flament, J.B.; Pochart, J.M.; Patey, M.; Marty, H.; Liehn, J.C. et al. (2008). SPECT/CT in localization of parathyroid adenoma or hyperplasia in patients with previous neck surgery. *Clinical Nuclear Medicine*, Vol.33, No.6 (Jun 2008), 394-397, ISSN: 0363-9762

Riss, P.; Kaczirek, K.; Heinz, G.; Bieglmayer, C. & Niederle, B. (2007). A "defined baseline" in PTH monitoring increases surgical success in patients with multiple gland disease. *Surgery*, Vol.142, No.3 (Sep 2007), pp. 398-404, ISSN: 0039-6060

Rubello, D.; Al-Nahhas, A.; Mariani, G.; Gross, M.D.; Rampin, L. & Pelizzo, M.R. (2006). Feasibility and longterm results of focused radioguided parathyroidectomy using a low 37 MBq (1 mCi) 99mTcsestamibi protocol. *International Seminars in Surgical Oncology*, Vol.3 (Sep 2006), p. 30, ISSN: 1477-7800

Rubello, D.; Casara, D.; Giannini, S.; Piotto, A.; de Carlo E.; Muzzio, P.C. & Pelizzo, M.R. (2003). Importance of radioguided minimally invasive parathyroidectomy using hand- help gammaprobe and low 99mTc MIBI dose. Technical considerations and long- term clinical result. *Quarterly Journal of Nuclear Medicine*, Vol.47, No.2 (Jun 2003), pp. 129-138, ISSN: 0392-0208

Rubello, D.; Casara, D. & Pelizzo, M.R. (2003). Symposium on parathyroid localization. Optimization of peroperative procedures. *Nuclear Medicine Communications*, Vol.24, No.2 (Feb 2003), pp. 133-140, ISSN: 0143-3636

Rubello, D.; Mariani, G.; Al-Nahhas, A. & Pelizzo, M.R. (2006). Minimally invasive radio-guided parathyroidectomy: long-term results with the "low 99mTc-sestamibi protocol". *Nuclear Medicine Communications*, Vol.27, No.9 (Sep 2006), pp 790-713, ISSN: 0143-3636

Scopinaro, F.; Di Luzio, E. & Pani, R. (1999). Sentinel lymph node biopsy in breast cancer: use of an imaging probe. In: Limouris, G.S.; Shukla, S.K. & Biersack, H.J., eds. Radionuclides for lymph nodes. Athens: Mediterranea Publishers, 1999; p. 60–5.

Sebag, F., Shen, W.; Brunaud. L.; Kebebew, E.; Duh, Q.Y. & Clark, O.H. (2003). Intraoperaive parathyroid hormone assay and parathyroid reoperations. *Surgery*, Vol.134, No.6 (Dec 2003), pp 1049-1055, ISSN: 0039-6060

Sidell, D.; Wang, J. & Sercarz, J. (2010). Spurious decline in intraoperative parathyroid hormone: false positives in parathyroid surgery. *American Journal of Otolaryngology*, Vol.31, No.6 (Nov-Dec 2010), pp. 479-481, ISSN 0196-0709

Siperstein, A.; Berber, E.; Mackey, R.; Alghoul, M.; Wagner, K. & Milas, M. (2004). Prospective evaluation of sestamibi scan, ultrasonography, and rapid PTH to predict the success of limited exploration for sporadic primary hyperparathyroidism. *Surgery*, Vol.136, No.4 (Oct 2004), pp 872-880, ISSN 0039-6060

Sitges-Serra, A.; Díaz-Aguirregoitia, F.J.; de la Quintana, A.; Gil-Sánchez, J.; Jimeno, J.; Prieto, R. et al. (2010). Weight difference between double parathyroid adenomas is the cause of false positive ioPTHi test after resection of the first lesion. *World Journal of Surgery*, Vol.34, No.6 (Jun 2010), pp 1337-1342, ISSN 0364-2313

Smith, N.; Magnuson, J.S.; Vidrine, D.M.; Kulbersh, B. & Peters, G.E. (2009). Minimally invasive parathyroidectomy. Use of intraoperative parathyroid assays after 2 preoperative localization studies. *Archives of Otolaryngology- Head & Neck Surgery*, Vol.135, No.11 (Nov 2009), pp 1108-1111, ISSN: 0886-4470

Solórzano, C.C.; Mendez, W.; Lew, J.I.; Rodgers, S.E.; Montano, R.; Carneiro-Pla, D.M. & Irvin, G.L. 3rd. (2008). Long-term outcome of patients with elevated parathyroid hormone levels after successful parathyroidectomy for sporadic primary hyperparathyroidism. *Archives of Surgery*, Vol.143, No.7 (Jul 2008), pp. 659-663, discussion p. 663, ISSN 0004-0010

Soluri A et al, inventors. Miniaturized gamma camera with very high spatial resolution. Italian patent RM97A000233, April 23,1997; US patent 6 242 744 B1, June 5, 2001.

Stratmann, S.L.; Kuhn, J.A.; Bell, M.S.; Preskitt, J.T.; O'Brien, J.C.; Gable, D.R.; Stephens, J.S. & McCarty, TM. (2002). Comparison of quick parathyroid assay for unilateral and multiglandular disease. *American Journal of Surgery*, Vol.184, No.6 (Dec 2002), pp. 578-581, ISSN 0002-9610

Sugg, S.L.; Krzywda, E.A.; Demeure, M.J. & Wilson, S.D. (2004). Detection of multiple gland primary hyperparathryidism in the era of minimally invasive parathyroidectomy. *Surgery*, Vol.136, No.6 (Dec 2004), pp. 1303-1309, ISSN: 0039-6060

Sugino, K.; Ito, K.; Nagahama, M.; Kitagawa, W.; Shibuya, H.; Ohkuwa, K. et al. (2010). Minimally invasive surgery for primary hyperparathryroidism with or without intraoperative parathyroid hormone monitoring. *Endocrine Journal*, Vol.57, No.11, pp. 953-958, ISSN 0918-8959

Takeyama, H.; Shioya, H.; Mori, Y.; Ogi, S.; Yamamoto, H.; Kaoto, N. et al. (2004). Usefulness of radio-guided surgery using Technetium-99m Methoxyisobutylisonitrile for primary and secondary Hyperparathyroidism. *World Journal of Surgery*, Vol.28, No.6 (Jun 2004), pp. 576-582, ISSN 0364-2313

Thompson, G.B. ; Grant, C.S. ; Perrier, N.D. et al. Reoperative (1999). Parathyroid surgery in the era of sestamibi scanning and intraoperative parathyroid hormone monitoring. *Archives of Surgery*, Vo.134, No.7 (Jul 1999), pp. 699-705, ISSN 0004-0010

Tibblin, S.; Bondeson, A.G. & Ljungberg, O. (1982). Unilateral parathyroidectomy in hyperparathyroidism due to single adenoma. *Annals of Surgery*, Vol.195, No.3 (March 1982), pp 245-252, ISSN 1528-1140

Ugur, Ö.; Bozkurt, M.F.; Hamaloglu, E.; Sokmensuer, C.; Etikan, I.; Ugur, Y. et al. (2004). Clinicopathologic and radiopharmacokinetic factors affecting gamma probe-guided parathyroidectomy. *Archives of Surgery*, Vol.139, No.11 (Nov 2004), pp 1175-1179, ISSN 0004-0010

Ugur, Ö.; Kara, P.Ö.; Bozkurt, M.F.; Hamaloglu, E.; Tezel, G.G.; Salanci, B.V, et al. (2006). In vivo characterisation of parathyroid lesions by use of gamma probe: comparison with ex vivo count method and frozen section results. *Otolaryngology-Head and Neck Surgery*, Vol.134, No.2 (Feb 2006), pp. 316-320, ISSN 0194-5998

Weigel, T.L.; Murphy, J.; Kabbani, L.; Ibele, A. & Chen, H. (2005). Radioguided thoracoscopic mediastinal parathyroidectomy with intraoperative parathyroid hormone testing. *The Annals of Thoracic Surgery*, Vol.80, No.4 (Oct 2005), pp. 1262–1265, ISSN 0003-4975

Yang, G.P.; Levine, S. & Weigel, R.J. (2001). A spike in parathyroid hormone during neck exploration may cause a false negative intraoperative assay result. *Archives of Surgery*, Vol.136, No.8 (Aug 2001), pp. 945-949, ISSN 0004-0010

Zettinig, G.; Kurtaran, A.; Prager, G.; Kaserer, K.; Dudczak, R. & Niederle, B. (2002). "Suppressed" double adenoma -a rare pitfall in minimally invasive parathyroidectomy. *Hormone Research.*, Vol.57, No.1-2, pp. 57-60, ISSN: 0301-0163

Part 3

Hyperparathyroidism and Dyalisis

5

Aluminum Overload: An Easily-Ignored Problem in Dialysis Patients with Hyperparathyroidism

Wei-Chih Kan[1,2], Chih-Chiang Chien[1,2], Yi-Hua Lu[1], Jyh-Chang Hwang[1], Shih-Bin Su[3,4] and Hsien-Yi Wang[1,5]
[1]*Department of Nephrology, Chi-Mei Medical Center, Tainan*
[2]*Chung Hwa University of Medical Technology, Tainan*
[3]*Department of Family Medicine, Chi-Mei Medical Center, Tainan*
[4]*Department of Biotechnology, Southern Taiwan University, Tainan*
[5]*Chia Nan University of Pharmacy and Science, Tainan*
Taiwan, R.O.C.

1. Introduction

Dialysis patients are at high risk for aluminum overload, especially patients with hyperparathyroidism, who may occasionally take aluminum-containing phosphate binders. Dialysis patients with aluminum overload may have various symptoms, such as general bone or muscle pain, iron-resistant anemia, hypercalcemia, and neurologic abnormalities, which are sometimes difficult to differentiate from clinical manifestations of hyperparathyroidism. Because of the different therapeutic strategies between aluminum overload and hyperparathyroidism, an overview of aluminum overload in dialysis patients with hyperparathyroidism is presented in the following sections.

2. Aluminum overload in dialysis patients

Dialysis patients are at high risk for aluminum overload (Jaffe, J.A. et al., 2005) because of long-term use of aluminum-containing phosphate binders (Humpfner, A. et al., 1993; Salusky, I.B., 2006), poor renal excretion of aluminum, and contact with aluminum-containing dialysate. Aluminum can be eliminated from dialysate by using reverse osmosis and deionization techniques. The dialysate concentration of aluminum is suggested to be maintained at <10 µg/L (Fernández-Martin, J.L. et al., 1998; National Kidney Foundation [NKF], 2003). Therefore, aluminum-containing phosphate binders had been documented as the predominant source of aluminum exposure in dialysis patients (Savory, J. et al., 1989; Slatopolsky, E., 1987). Because of multiple systemic aluminum-related complications, reducing the exposure of dialysis patients to aluminum by substituting calcium- and other non-aluminum-based phosphate binders is a well-known concept. However, some patients with refractory hyperphosphatemia or calcium-induced hypercalcemia still require aluminum therapy (NKF, 2003). While aluminum-based phosphate binders used as short-term therapy are suggested by the Kidney Disease Outcomes Quality Initiative (K/DOQI) guidelines, these medications are prohibited in some countries (Koiwa, F., & Sato, Y., 2009). Non-calcium and non-aluminum phosphate binders (such as sevelamer hydrochloride and lanthanum carbonate) are suggested as substitutes. However, these newly developed medications have not become popular in many countries because of their high cost (Koiwa, F. & Sato, Y., 2009). In addition, the source of aluminum may contribute to extra aluminum intake from other medications (Bohrer, D. et al., 2009). Therefore, aluminum overload is still a potential problem in the dialysis population.

2.1 Frequency of aluminum overload

The declining exposure of aluminum-containing dialysate and medications with commonly use of high flux dialyzers has resulted in a low incidence of abnormal aluminum levels in current dialysis patients (Cannata-Andía, J.B. & Fernández-Martín, J.L., 2002). In one retrospective study on more than 43,000 dialysis patients, 2.5% of the patients had elevated serum aluminum levels (>50 μg/L) that significantly declined year by year (Jaffe, J.A. et al., 2005). However, the prevalence of aluminum overload might be higher in countries that still commonly used aluminum-containing phosphate binders (Kan, W.C. et al., 2010).

2.2 Clinical manifestations of aluminum overload

Aluminum can accumulate in many human organs; this accumulation has been implicated in various diseases, including dialysis encephalopathy, aluminum-induced bone disease (such as osteomalacia), hypercalcemia, and iron-resistant microcytic anemia (NKF, 2003; Berlyne, G.M. et al., 1970, 1972; Sherrard, D.J., 1974; Alfrey, A.C. et al., 1976, 1987; Ward, M.K. et al., 1978; Parkinson, I.S. et al., 1979; Drüeke T., 1980; Hewitt, C.D. et al., 1990). (Summary of Aluminum-related disorders: Features, Causes, and Considerations for therapy, http://www.kidney.org/professionals/kdoqi/guidelines_bone/images/table311.jpg)

2.2.1 Dialysis encephalopathy

Dialysis encephalopathy is usually a slowly progressive disorder with symptoms appearing after a patient has undergone dialysis for 1 year or even longer. Increased aluminum is found in the brain tissue of affected patients (Alfrey, A.C. et al., 1976). It is characterized by myoclonic jerks, mental changes, speech disturbances, visual or auditory hallucinations, paranoid behaviors, and even seizures. These neurologic abnormalities maybe fluctuate and often worsen temporarily after hemodialysis. The typical electroencephalographic (EEG) findings differ from the generalized slow wave with other causes of metabolic encephalopathy (Hughes, J.R. & Schreeder, M.T., 1980). However, due to its insidious progression, diagnosing these neurological disorders depends on clinical observation and suspicion, the finding of elevated plasma aluminum levels, and associated EEG features. New cases of dialysis encephalopathy disappeared after the initiation of water purification in 1979, and no more new cases have been reported in the developed countries since then (NKF, 2003).

2.2.2 Aluminum-induced bone disease

Aluminum can affect normal bone formation via several mechanisms. First, it interferes with mineralization of the matrix by forming crystals to compete for the site of calcium deposition, and it inhibits the activity of osteoblasts, both of which impair bone-building (Jeffery, E.H. et al., 1996). Second, it binds in the parathyroid gland, which inhibits the normal secretion of parathyroid hormone (PTH) (Cannata, J.B. et al., 1988), and it impairs PTH synthesis at the transcriptional level (Díaz-Corte, C. et al., 2001). Because of abnormal bone formation, osteomalacia is the most frequently seen aluminum-induced bone disease, but its prevalence is reported to have markedly decreased after reduced exposure to aluminum (NKF, 2003). Osteomalacia is characterized by a low rate of bone turnover, a decreased number of bone-forming and bone-resorbing cells, and an increased volume of unmineralized bone (Delmez, J.A. & Slatopolsky, E., 1992; Slatopolsky, E., 1987). In addition, because of its potential to excessively suppress PTH, aluminum overload may cause adynamic bone disease in a minority of cases.

2.2.3 Anemia

Aluminum can also affect normal hemopoietic processes via several mechanisms. First, it impairs intestinal absorption, serum transport, and cellular uptake of iron, because aluminum and iron share a common absorption pathway and, in the serum, they are transported on the same carriers in humans (Kausz, A.T. et al., 1999). These carriers include large proteins (such as transferrin and albumin) and small molecules (such as citrate and phosphate). In several animal and human studies, a significant negative correlation was found between aluminum load and iron transferrin saturation (Cannata, J.B. et al., 1991), and additional reductions in the use of aluminum-containing medications led to significant increases in hemoglobin and reductions in the need for intravenous iron supplementation in hemodialysis patients (Cannata, J.B. et al., 1983a). Second, aluminum may induce resistance to the hematopoietic effects of recombinant human erythropoietin (rHuEPO) in both rats and dialysis patients (Drüeke, T.B., 1990; Losekann, A. et al., 1990). Therefore, dialysis patients with an obvious aluminum overload may need larger doses of rHuEPO to overcome this resistance, which significantly increases the cost of patient care.

2.2.4 Hypercalcemia

Aluminum-related bone disease may cause hypercalcemia (Norris, K.C. et al., 1985). In a rat study, aluminum changed the relationships between serum PTH, calcium, and phosphorus (Felsenfeld, A.J. et al., 1993). In a study of 25 patients on continuous ambulatory peritoneal dialysis (Cannata, J.B. et al., 1983b) who had accidentally been exposed to high level of aluminum in the dialysate for a month, serum calcium levels significantly increased from 2.27 to 2.44 mmol/L, while serum PTH levels declined from 744 to 580 ng/L. In another study of hemodialysis patients (Cannata, J.B. et al., 1983c), a high serum aluminum level was strongly associated with hypercalcemia and low serum PTH level. Therefore, the suspicion of aluminum overload should be kept in mind in the patient who does not have obvious elevations in serum intact PTH (e.g., less than 500 pg/mL) or who is not taking vitamin D therapy (NKF, 2003).

2.3 Screening and diagnosis for aluminum overload

A histological examination of bone biopsy specimens is still considered the gold standard for diagnosing dialysis patients with an aluminum overload. Biopsies, however, are invasive and expensive. Therefore, several studies have reported their efforts to develop less invasive diagnostic methods of diagnosing aluminum overload (Milliner, D.S. et al., 1984). Serum aluminum measurements are of limited value due to its high tissue accumulation. However, aluminum overload is unlikely in dialysis patients with baseline serum aluminum concentrations (without desferrioxamine (DFO) "stimulation") less than 20 μg/L (NKF, 2003). In one study, 50 dialysis patients undergoing bone biopsy seemed distinguishable, after a DFO infusion test, from those with a positive bone aluminum stain by an increase in serum aluminum and a relatively high serum iPTH level (McCarthy, J.T. et al., 1990). In another prospective study of 445 dialysis patients to evaluate noninvasive tests that combined the results of intact parathyroid hormone (iPTH) and DFO tests (Pei, Y. et al., 1992), the test were useful for predicting aluminum-related bone disease in dialysis patients using aluminum-based binders. However, they yielded a high incidence of false-negatives and low-sensitivity results after these patients had discontinued aluminum-based binders for more than 6 months. According to the present consensus, the DFO test affords a non-invasive method to identify patients with an increased body burden of aluminum (NKF, 2003) (Evaluation of aluminum-related disorders: considerations for DFO test and subsequent DFO treatment, http://www.kidney.org/professionals/kdoqi/guidelines_bone/Images/Algorithm7L.jpg).

2.4 Treatment

In addition to dialysis modalities, the K/DOQI guideline (NKF, 2003) also recommends DFO to treat dialysis patients with an aluminum overload. However, DFO has side effects of its own (Cronin, R.E. & Henrich, W.L., 2006), such as itchy skin, nausea, myalgia, and neurotoxicity (McCauley, J. & Sorkin, M.I., 1989). Although most of these side effects are mild and reversible, some rare and severe or even life-threatening side effects are possible, especially anaphylactic shock and mucormycosis (Boelaert, J.R. et al., 1991, 1993). Because of the common side effects of DFO, doses of 20-40 mg/kg of body weight (Bene, C. et al., 1989; Cases, A. et al., 1988; Pengloan, J. et al., 1987) have been abandoned. The toxicity of DFO is dose-dependent; thus, many studies (Barata, J.D. et al., 1996; D'Haese, P.C. et al., 1995; Janssen, M.J. & van Boven, W.P., 1996) were designed to find the optimal dose for aluminum overload treatment. According to the K/DOQI clinical practice guideline (NKF, 2003), the DFO standard dose is 5 mg/kg of body weight (DFO treatment, http://www.kidney.org/professionals/kdoqi/guidelines_bone/Images/Algorithm9L.jpg). Furthermore, several pharmacokinetic and small-scale, short-term studies (Canteros, A. et al., 1998; Jorge, C. et al., 1999) found that even doses lower than 5 mg/kg were as efficacious as the standard 5 mg/kg dose, but clinical trials verifying its efficacy at lower doses are lacking. Therefore, we compared the response to 2 months of treatment with the standard dose (5 mg/kg) versus a lower dose (2.5 mg/kg) of DFO in dialysis patients with aluminum overload. Both treatment groups showed similar therapeutic effects, there were relatively fewer side effects in the 2.5-mg/kg group (Kan, W.C. et al., 2010).

3. Managing aluminum overload in dialysis patients with hyperparathyroidism

In patients with hyperparathyroidism, calcium-based phosphate binders are always unsuitable because of the frequently associated symptoms of hypercalcemia. Therefore, aluminum-based binders were used, which created a high risk of aluminum overload. Because PTH can protect against aluminum deposition at the mineralization front, perhaps by increasing bone turnover (Slatopolsky, E., 1987), the symptoms of aluminum-related bone diseases may be "masked" in dialysis patients with hyperparathyroidism. However, this "protection" will disappear in patients who have undergone a parathyroidectomy (PTX), because lowered PTH levels will accelerate bone aluminum deposition (Slatopolsky, E., 1987). Therefore, it is generally suggested that aluminum bone disease be excluded before PTX. Similarly, medical treatment of hyperparathyroidism with active Vitamin D3 (calcitriol) also may accelerate aluminum bone disease. In addition, the risk of aluminum bone disease is greater in diabetics (Andress, D.L. et al., 1987; Pei, Y. et al., 1993), which may be related to a lower bone turnover rate, which has been reported in type 1 diabetics before the onset of clinical renal disease (Andress, D.L. et al., 1987; Vincenti, F. et al., 1984). Therefore, because of the sometimes similar clinical manifestations of hyperparathyroidism and aluminum overload, physicians treating dialysis patients with hyperparathyroidism should consider the possibility of concurrent aluminum problems, especially in high-risk diabetic patients.

The side effects of DFO are dose-dependent and potentially life-threatening. Although the standard dose for aluminum overload is 5 mg/kg/week for a total of 8 weeks, there are still reports of fatal mucormycosis on such a regimen (Petrikkos, G. & Drogari-Apiranthitou, M., 2011). A lower dose of DFO, if it offers good efficacy with fewer side effects, may be promising for managing such complicated patients (Kan, W.C. et al., 2010).

4. Conclusion

Although the prevalence of aluminum overload in dialysis patients is decreasing, it is still an insidious problem worldwide, especially in these dialysis patients still often exposed to aluminum-containing medications. In these patients with hyperparathyroidism, calcium- and aluminum-based binders are not suitable for long-term use (particularly for patients on concurrent vitamin D therapy). Therefore, in these particular patients, especially those with a history of aluminum-containing medications or water exposure, possible concurrent aluminum overload should be kept in mind before medical or surgical intervention. Otherwise, aluminum-related bone disease will be aggravated after treatments. Therefore, several non-calcium, non-aluminum phosphate binders (such as sevelamer hydrochloride and lanthanum carbonate) are suggested despite the high cost and consequent unpopularity of these newly developed medications.

5. Acknowledgment

Sincerely thankful to Miss Hui-Li Hsiao, the Matron of the Dialysis Center in Chi-Mei Medical Center, and all the staff nurses, whose full support and encouragement enabled us to complete the related studies.

6. References

Alfrey, A.C., LeGendre, G.R., Kaehny, W.D. (1976). The dialysis encephalopathy syndrome. Possible aluminum intoxication. *N Engl J Med.*, Vol. 294, pp. 184–188, ISSN 1533-4406

Alfrey A.C. (1987). Aluminum metabolism and toxicity in uremia. *J UOEH.*, Vol. 9, Suppl, pp. 123–132, ISSN 0387-821X

Andress, D.L., Kopp, J.B., Maloney, N.A., Coburn, J.W., Sherrard, D.J. (1987). Early deposition of aluminum in bone in diabetic patients on hemodialysis. *N Engl J Med.*, Vol. 316, No. 6, pp. 292-296, ISSN 1533-4406

Barata, J.D., D'Haese, P.C., Pires, C., Lamberts, L.V., Simões, J., De Broe, M.E. (1996). Low-dose (5 mg/kg) desferrioxamine treatment in acutely aluminium-intoxicated haemodialysis patients using two drug administration schedules. *Nephrol Dial Transplant.*, Vol. 11, No. 1, pp. 125-132, ISSN 1460-2385

Bene, C., Manzler, A., Bene, D., Kranias, G. (1989). Irreversible ocular toxicity from single "challenge" dose of deferoxamine. *Clin Nephrol.*, Vol. 31, No. 1, pp. 45-48, ISSN 0301-0430

Berlyne, G.M., Pest, D., Ben-Ari, J., Weinberger, J., Stern, M., Gilmore, G.R., Levine, R. (1970). Hyperaluminaemia from aluminum resins in renal failure. *Lancet,* Vol. 296, No. 7671, pp. 494–496, ISSN 1474-547X

Berlyne, G.M., Ben-Ari, J., Knopf, E., Yagil, R., Weinberger, G., Danovitch, G.M. (1972). Aluminium toxicity in rats. *Lancet,* Vol. 299, No. 7750, pp. 564–568, ISSN 1474-547X

Boelaert, J.R., Fenves, A.Z., Coburn, J.W. (1991). Deferoxamine therapy and mucormycosis in dialysis patients: Report of an international registry. *Am J Kidney Dis.,* Vol. 18, pp. 660-667, ISSN 1523-6838

Boelaert, J.R., de Locht, M., Van Cutsem, J., Kerrels, V., Cantinieaux, B., Verdonck, A., Van Landuyt, H.W., Schneider, YJ. (1993). Mucormycosis during deferoxamine therapy is a siderophore-mediated infection. In vitro and in vivo animal studies. *J Clin Invest.,* Vol. 91, No. 5, pp. 1979-1986

Bohrer, D., Bertagnolli, D.C., de Oliveira, S.M., do Nascimento, P.C., de Carvalho, L.M., Garcia, S.C., Arantes, L.C., Barros, E.J. (2009). Role of medication in the level of aluminium in the blood of chronic renal patients. *Nephrol Dial Transplant.,* Vol. 24, pp. 1277-1281, ISSN 1460-2385

Cannata, J.B., Ruiz Alegria, P., Cuesta, M.V., Herrera, J., Peral, V. (1983). Influence of aluminium hydroxide intake on haemoglobin concentrations and blood transfusion requirements in haemodialysis patients. *Proc Eur Dial Transplant Assoc.,* Vol. 20, pp. 719–724, ISSN 0308-9401

Cannata, J.B., Junor, B.J., Briggs, J.D., Fell, G.S., Beastall, G. Effect of acute aluminium overload on calcium and parathyroid-hormone metabolism. (1983). *Lancet,* Vol. 321, No. 8323, pp. 501–503, ISSN 1474-547X

Cannata, J.B., Briggs, J.D., Junor, B.J., Beastall, G., Fell, G.S. (1983). The influence of aluminium on parathyroid hormone levels in haemodialysis patients. *Proc Eur Dial Transplant Assoc.,* Vol. 19, pp. 244–247, ISSN 0308-9401

Cannata, J.B., Diaz Lopez, J.B., Fernandez Menendez, M.J., Virgos, M.J. (1988). The parathyroid gland and aluminum overload: an overview. *Contrib Nephrol.,* Vol. 64, pp. 113–119, ISSN 0302-5144

Cannata, J.B., Fernández-Soto, I., Fernández-Menendez, M.J., Fernández-Martín, J.L., McGregor, S.J., Brock, J.H., Halls, D. (1991). Role of iron metabolism in absorption and cellular uptake of aluminum. *Kidney Int.,* Vol. 39, No. 4, pp. 799–803, ISSN 1523-1755

Cannata, J.B., and Fernández-Martín, J.L. (2002). The clinical impact of aluminium overload in renal failure. *Nephrol Dial Transplant.,* Vol. 17, Suppl 2, pp. 9-12.

Canteros, A., Díaz-Corte, C., Fernández-Martín, J.L., Gago, E., Fernández-Merayo, C., Cannata, J. (1998). Ultrafiltrable aluminium after very low doses of desferrioxamine. *Nephrol Dial Transplant.,* Vol. 13, No. 6, pp. 1538-1542, ISSN 1460-2385

Cases, A., Kelly, J., Sabater, J., Campistol, J.M., Torras, A., Montoliu, J., López, I., Revert, L. (1988). Acute visual and auditory neurotoxicity in patients with end-stage renal disease receiving desferrioxamine. *Clin Nephrol.,* Vol. 29, No. 4, pp. 176-178, ISSN 0301-0430

Cronin, R.E., and Henrich, W.L. (2006). Aluminum toxicity in end-stage renal disease. *In: UpToDate, Rose, BD (Ed), UpToDate, Waltham, MA,* ISSN 0301-5718

Delmez, J.A., and Slatopolsky, E. (1992). Hyperphosphatemia: its consequences and treatment in patients with chronic renal disease. *Am J Kidney Dis.,* Vol. 19, No. 4, pp. 303-317, ISSN 1523-6838

D'Haese, P.C., Couttenye, M.M., Goodman, W.G., Lemoniatou, E., Digenis, P., Sotornik, I., Fagalde, A., Barsoum, R.S., Lamberts, L.V., De Broe, M.E. (1995). Use of the low-dose desferrioxamine test to diagnose and differentiate between patients with aluminium-related bone disease, increased risk for aluminium toxicity, or aluminium overload. *Nephrol Dial Transplant.*, Vol. 10, No. 10, pp. 1874-1884, ISSN 1460-2385

Díaz-Corte, C., Fernández-Martín, J.L., Barreto, S., Gómez, C., Fernández-Coto, T., Braga, S., Cannata, J.B. (2001). Effect of aluminium load on parathyroid hormone synthesis. *Nephrol Dial Transplant.*, Vol. 16, pp. 742–745, ISSN 1460-2385

Drüeke T. (1980). Dialysis osteomalacia and aluminum intoxication. *Nephron* Vol. 26, pp. 207–210, ISSN 1660-2110

Drüeke, T.B. (1990). Resistance to recombinant human erythropoietin in hemodialysis patients. *Am J Nephrol.*, Vol. 10, Suppl. 2, pp. 34–39, ISSN 1421-9670

Felsenfeld, A.J., Machado, L., Bover, J., Trinidad, P., Rodriguez, M. (1993). Effect of aluminium on the development of hyperparathyroidism and bone disease in the azotaemic rat. *Nephrol Dial Transplant.*, Vol. 8, No. 4, pp. 325–334, ISSN 1460-2385

Fernández-Martin, J.L., Canteros, A., Serrano, M., Gonzalez-Carcedo, A., Diaz-Corte, C., Cannata, J.B. (1998). Prevention of aluminium exposure through dialysis fluids. Analysis of changes in the last 8 years. *Nephrol Dial Transplant.*, Vol. 13, Suppl 3, pp. 78–81, ISSN 1460-2385

Hewitt, C.D., Savory, J., Wills, M.R. (1990). Aspects of aluminum toxicity. *Clin Lab Med.*, Vol. 10, pp. 403–422, ISSN 1437-4331

Hughes, J.R., and Schreeder, M.T. (1980). EEG in dialysis encephalopathy. *Neurology.*, Vol. 30, No. 11, pp. 1148-1154, ISSN 1526-632X

Humpfner, A., Hummel, S., Schultz, W. (1993). Diagnosis and therapeutic approaches to aluminum overload in dialysed patients--representative study questionnaire in West German dialysis units in 1989-1990. *Nephrol Dial Transplant.*, Vol. 8, Suppl. 1, pp. S51-S54, ISSN 1460-2385

Jaffe, J.A., Liftman, C., Glickman, J.D. (2005). Frequency of elevated serum aluminum levels in adult dialysis patients. *Am J Kidney Dis.*, Vol. 46, No. 2, pp. 316-319, ISSN 1523-6838

Jeffery, E.H., Abreo, K., Burgess, E., Cannata, J., Greger, J.L. (1996). Systemic aluminum toxicity: effects on bone, hematopoietic tissue, and kidney. *J Toxicol Environ Health.*, Vol. 48, pp. 649–665, ISSN 0098-4108

Janssen, M.J., and van Boven, W.P. (1996). Efficacy of low-dose desferrioxamine for the estimation of aluminium overload in haemodialysis patients. *Pharm World Sci.*, Vol. 18, pp. 187-191, ISSN 1573-739X

Jorge, C., Gil, C., Possante, M., Catarino, M.C., Cruz, A., Andrade, R., Teixeira, R., Santos, N., Ferreira, A. (1999). Use of a desferrioxamine "microdose" to chelate aluminum in hemodialysis patients. *Clin Nephrol.*, Vol. 52, No. 5, pp. 335-336, ISSN 0301-0430

Kan, W.C., Chien, C.C., Wu, C.C., Su, S.B., Hwang, J.C., Wang, H.Y. (2010). Comparison of low-dose deferoxamine versus standard-dose deferoxamine for treatment of aluminium overload among haemodialysis patients. *Nephrol Dial Transplant.*, Vol. 25, No. 5, pp. 1604-1608, ISSN 1460-2385

Kausz, A.T., Antonsen, J.E., Hercz, G., Pei, Y., Weiss, N.S., Emerson, S., Sherrard, D.J. (1999). Screening plasma aluminum levels in relation to aluminum bone disease among asymptomatic dialysis patients. *Am J Kidney Dis.*, Vol. 34, No. 4, pp. 688-693, ISSN 1523-6838

Koiwa, F., and Sato, Y. (2009). Chemistry and history of phosphate binder. *Clin Calcium.*, Vol. 19, pp. 198-204, ISSN 0917-5857

Losekann, A., Ureña, P., Khiraoui, F., Casadevall, N., Zins, B., Bererhi, L., Zingraff, J., Bourdon, R., Drüeke, T. (1990). Aluminium intoxication in the rat induces partial resistance to the effect of recombinant human erythropoietin. *Nephrol Dial Transplant.*, Vol. 5, No. 4, pp. 258–263, ISSN 1460-2385

McCarthy, J.T., Milliner, D.S., Johnson, W.J. (1990). Clinical experience with desferrioxamine in dialysis patients with aluminium toxicity. *Q J Med.*, Vol. 74, pp. 257-276, ISSN 1460-2393

McCauley, J., and Sorkin, M.I. (1989). Exacerbation of aluminum encephalopathy after treatment with desferrioxamine. *Nephrol Dial Transplant.*, Vol. 4, No. 2, pp. 110-114, ISSN 1460-2385

Milliner, D.S., Nebeker, H.G., Ott, S.M., Andress, D.L., Sherrard, D.J., Alfrey, A.C., Slatopolsky, E.A., Coburn, J.W. (1984). Use of the deferoxamine infusion test in the diagnosis of aluminum-related osteodystrophy. *Ann Intern Med.*, Vol. 101, No. 6, pp. 775-779, ISSN 1539-3704

National Kidney Foundation. K/DOQI clinical practice guidelines for bone metabolism and disease in chronic kidney disease. (2003). *Am J Kidney Dis.*, Vol. 42, pp. S108-S122, ISSN 1523-6838

Norris, K.C., Crooks, P.W., Nebeker, H.G., Hercz, G., Milliner, D.S., Gerszi, K., Slatopolsky, E., Andress, D.L., Sherrard, D.J., Coburn J.W. (1985). Clinical and laboratory features of aluminum-related bone disease: Differences between sporadic and "epidemic" forms of the syndrome. *Am J Kidney Dis.*, Vol. 6, pp. 342-347, ISSN 1523-6838

Parkinson, I.S., Ward, M.K., Feest, T.G., Fawcett, R.W., Kerr, D.N. (1979). Fracturing dialysis osteodystrophy and dialysis encephalopathy. An epidemiological survey. *Lancet*, Vol. 313, No. 8113, pp. 406–409, ISSN 1474-547X

Pei, Y., Hercz, G., Greenwood, C., Sherrard, D., Segre, G., Manuel, A., Saiphoo, C., Fenton, S. (1992). Non-invasive prediction of aluminum bone disease in hemo- and peritoneal dialysis patients. *Kidney Int.*, Vol. 41, No. 5, pp. 1374–1382, ISSN 1523-1755

Pei, Y., Hercz, G., Greenwood, C., Segre, G., Manuel, A., Saiphoo, C., Fenton, S., Sherrard, D. (1993). Renal osteodystrophy in diabetic patients. *Kidney Int.*, Vol. 44, No. 1, pp. 159-164, ISSN 1523-1755

Pengloan, J., Dantal, J., Rossazza, C., Abazza, M., Nivet, H. (1987). Ocular toxicity after a single intravenous dose of desferrioxamine in 2 hemodialyzed patients. *Nephron*, Vol. 46, No. 2, pp. 211-212, ISSN 1660-2110

Petrikkos, G., and Drogari-Apiranthitou, M. (2011). Zygomycosis in immunocompromised non-haematological patients. *Mediterr J Hematol Infect Dis.*, Vol. 3, No. 1, e2011012, ISSN 2035-3006

Salusky, I.B. (2006). A new era in phosphate binder therapy: What are the options? *Kidney Int.*, Vol. 105, pp. S10-S15, ISSN 1523-1755

Savory, J., Berlin, A., Courtoux, C., Yeoman, B., Wills, M. (1989). Summary report of an international workshop on "The role of biological monitoring in the prevention of aluminum toxicity in man: Aluminum analysis in biological fluids." *Ann Clin Lab Sci.*, Vol. 13, pp. 444-451, ISSN 1550-8080

Sherrard, D.J. (1974). Letter: the myth of aluminum toxicity. *N Engl J Med.*, Vol. 290, pp. 750, ISSN 1533-4406

Slatopolsky, E. (1987). The interaction of parathyroid hormone and aluminum in renal osteodystrophy. *Kidney Int.*, Vol. 31, No. 3, pp. 842-854, ISSN 1523-1755

Vincenti, F., Arnaud, S.B., Recker, R., Genant, H., Amend, W.J., Jr., Feduska, N.J., Salvatierra, O., Jr. (1984). Parathyroid and bone response of the diabetic patient to uremia. *Kidney Int.*, Vol. 25, No. 4, pp. 677-682, ISSN 1523-1755

Ward, M.K., Ellis, H.A., Feest, T.G., Parkinson, I.S., Kerr, D.N. (1978). Osteomalacic dialysis osteodystrophy: evidence for a water-borne aetiological agent, probably aluminium. *Lancet*, Vol. 311, No. 8069, pp. 841–845, ISSN 1474-547X

6

Hyperparathyroidism in Hemodialyzed Patients – Relation to Melatonin and Reproductive Hormones Before and After Parathyroidectomy

Radmila Kancheva et al*
Institute of Endocrinology, Prague
Czech Republic

1. Introduction

Currently there is considerable interest generated about the interaction of parathyroid glands, possible role of melatonin and reproductive hormones on bone metabolism. In hemodialyzed (HD) patients with hyperparathyroidism (HPT) the melatonin concentrations are affected, but still not well studied. It has been also pointed out that the removal of the pineal gland or administration of its extracts produces alterations in the morphology and hormone secretion of the parathyroid glands (Kiss et al., 1969; Shoumura et al., 1992). On the other hand, parathyroidectomy (PTX) leads to sleep disturbances (Chou et al., 2005).

Renal diseases and hemodialysis are accompanied by profound changes in the mineral metabolism (Block et al., 2004; Hutchison et al., 1993). These changes are often associated with large variation of HPT. It is also well known that secondary HPT is common in chronic kidney disease patients (Chan et al, 2010; Rudser et al., 2007; Tominaga et al., 2001). Changes in the levels of gonadal steroids also occur in elderly patients, particularly in HD ones. However, it is not fully elucidated if the replacement steroid therapy influences parathyroid hormone responsiveness to hypercalcemia.

In HD patients melatonin disturbances are known to occur (Kancheva et al., 2008; Koch et al., 2009a, 2009b). In addition, patients with end-stage renal disease suffer from a number of related disorders (Koch et al., 2010a; Lüdemann et al., 2001; Young et al., 2005) including endocrine abnormalities, psychiatric disorders and impairment of sleep parameters. It seems

* Ivana Zofkova[1], Martin Hill[1], Sylvie Dusilova-Sulkova[2], Ludmila Kancheva[1], Sven Röjdmark[3], Antonin Parizek[4], Michaela Duskova[1], Zoltan Paluch[5], Veronika Cirmanova[1] and Luboslav Starka[1]
[1]*Institute of Endocrinology, Prague*
[2]*Nephrology Clinic, Institute of Clinical and Experimental Medicine, Prague*
[3]*Department of Internal Medicne, Endocrinology Section, Södersjukhuset, Stockholm*
[4]*Department of Obstetrics and Gynecology,*
First Medical Faculty Charles University Prague
[5]*Department of Medicine I, Thomayer University Hospital, Prague*
[1,2,4,5,6]*Czech Republic*
[3]*Sweden*

that there is a difference between conventional daytime HD and nocturnal HD patients. While in nocturnal HD patients nocturnal melatonin rise is noticed, in daytime and peritoneal dialysis patients such rise is absent (Koch et al., 2010b). Some data also suggest that melatonin (or pineal extract) is involved directly in the changes of the ultrastructure of the hamsters' parathyroid glands and in the amount of pro-secretory cell granules (Chan et al., 1991). Animal data indicated that the pineal melatonin is involved in the regulation of calcium and phosphate metabolism by stimulating the activity of the parathyroid glands and by inhibiting calcitonin release. Calcium decline is connected with parathyroid hormone secretion increase and *vice versa*.

There are reports of the direct effects of melatonin on calcium metabolism (Csaba & Baráth, 1974; Csaba & Bókay, 1977) and more recent findings of melatonin effects on the development of osteopenia associated with loss of gonadal function and senescence (Cardinali et al, 2003; Heaton & Morales, 2001; Ostrowska et al., 2010; Sandyk et al., 1922). Melatonin has an impact in the occurrence of the bone disorders and some authors have suggested that the hormone could be used as diagnostic and even therapeutic tool (Sánchez-Barceló et al., 2010). It should be mentioned that melatonin influences bone tissue metabolism and a possible mechanism might involve regulation of calciotropic and gonadal hormones (Heaton & Morales, 2001; Ladizesky et al., 2003). Long term melatonin administration is rather inhibitory on parathyroid function and bone metabolism.

The levels of parathyroid hormone and the gonadal hormones are affected by the so termed chronic kidney disease-mineral and bone disorders. (Doumouchtsis et al., 2008; Gal-Moscovici & Sprague, 2007; Gardham et al., 2010; Hamada & Fukagawa, 2009; Moe et al., 2007). Recent studies of androgens on bone physiology and mineral metabolism at cellular level in animal models and humans revealed that androgen steroids influence bone mass, age related bone loss and the occurrence of fractures, especially in elderly men (Ebeling, 1998, 2010.; Lindberg et al., 2005; Vanderschueren et al., 2004) Nevertheless, the specific role of androgens in bone metabolism and skeletal maintenance in men and women is still not fully understood.

The major circulating androgen in men is testosterone. In peripheral tissues it is converted by 5a-reductase to 5a-dihydrotestosterone (DHT). Androgens have anti-osteoporotic effect via direct interaction with androgen receptors, as well as effect mediated by estrogen receptors after aromatization to estradiol (Ashida et al., 2010). In the same time the pivot role of estrogens on bone formation recently has also been underlined (Leder et al., 2003; Riggs et al., 2002). The relative contribution of sex steroids on bone health and turnover remains still unclear, particularly in HD patients with HPT, because gonadal hormones concentrations are usually affected in chronic renal failure (Doumouchtsis et al., 2008, 2009). Cytochrome P450 enzyme aromatase system is a key component converting adrenal and testicular C19 steroids into C18 steroids. Experimental studies and some clinical observations have directly pointed out the importance of aromatization of androgens into estrogens (Gennari et al., 2004; Nuti et al., 2007). A priming estrogen effect on androgen acting on bone metabolism level is not excluded (Rochira et al., 2007; Zirilli et al., 2008).

Follicle stimulating hormone (FSH) and luteinizing hormone (LH) are suspected to be negatively associated with bone mineral status (Doumouchtsis et al., 2008). In pregnant rats PTX decreases GnRH (gonadotropin releasing hormone)-stimulated release of LH and FSH in their offspring (Fujii et al., 1986). Allan et al. (2010) demonstrated that FSH has dose-dependent anabolic effects on bone via an ovary-dependent mechanism, which is independent of LH activity, and does not involve direct FSH actions on bone cells. According to Kovács et al. (1994) after PTX in postmenopausal women the stimulated by GnRH secretion of FSH was significantly decreased while the decrease of LH secretion was not significant. The relative contribution and relationships among testosterone, LH, FSH and parathyroid hormone in HD patients with HPT are still not well known and deserve further elucidation.

2. Relationship between parathyroidectomy, calcium, phosphate and melatonin levels in hemodialyzed patients

In HD patients several disturbances are known to occur. Among them are the changes of melatonin secretion and its proposed effects on the levels of calcitonin and parathyroid hormone. Indeed, after pinealectomy functional changes in parathyroid glands take place. It could be expected that the elevated levels of calcium in HPT patients on HD and subsequently their decrease after PTX might influence the plasma concentrations of melatonin.

Nine HD patients with HPT participated in the study. Two profiles of nocturnal melatonin and parathyroid hormone were performed on each participant, i.e. before and 1-3 months after PTX. In addition, serum levels of calcium and phosphate were followed twice - before and after the operation. Melatonin concentrations were determined by the method of Fraser et al. (1983), intact parathyroid hormone - with a commercial kit from Nichols Institute, San Juan Capistrano, CA, USA and serum minerals by Merck Autoanalyzer.

Due to the non-Gaussian data distribution the variables of nocturnal profiles of melatonin and parathyroid hormone were treated by a power transformation to attain symmetric distribution and constant variance (Meloun et al, 2000, 2002).

Nocturnal profiles of melatonin in HD patients before and after PTX showed significant time dependence (F-ratio=3.14, $p<0.002$, ANOVA) which was much weaker when the effect of PTX was taken into account. The dependence is presented on Figure 1. It could be seen that the operation resulted in a significant increase in nocturnal melatonin concentrations (F-ratio=11.2, $p<0.002$, ANOVA).

As expected, the PTX was followed by radical parathyroid hormone decrease (F-ratio=682, $p<0.0001$, ANOVA), which showed no nocturnal variation both before and after the PTX - Figure 2.

Calcium and phosphate levels were measured before and after the PTX each time at the beginning of blood sampling. Individual mineral levels are presented on Figure 3. Calcium concentrations significantly decreased ($p<0.001$, Student's paired t- test) after the operation while phosphate levels increased ($p<0.05$, Wilcoxon's robust paired t-test).

The detail parameters of the investigated hormones and minerals before and after the operation and their differences are presented in Table 1.

Despite of the nocturnal melatonin increase in patients after parathyroidectomy Kancheva et al (2008) found that the patients return to more physiological way of melatonin secretion, i.e. with lower baseline levels and a relative higher further increase. It is difficult to speculate about the possible reasons for the occurrence of the aforementioned described phenomenon as the number of participants in the study was limited.

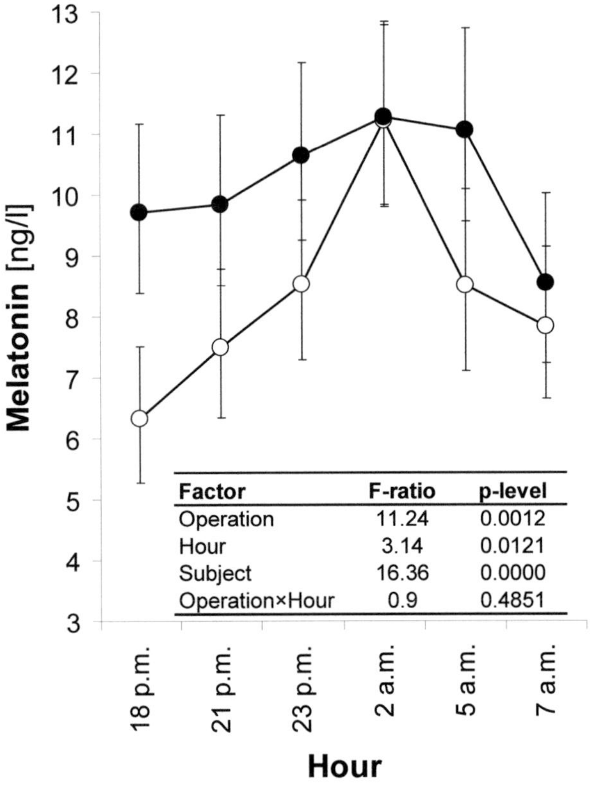

Fig. 1. Nocturnal profiles of melatonin in hemodialyzed patients before and after parathyroidectomy evaluated by repeated measures ANOVA consisting of Operation (before, after) and Hour within-subject factors, subject factor, and Operation × Hour interaction. The empty and full circles represent re-transformed mean melatonin levels with their 95% confidence intervals for individual hours of the trial before and after parathyroidectomy, respectively.

In patients with end-stage renal disease mineral metabolism disturbances are usual outcome of the disease (Lamb et al, 2007). Elevation in serum calcium levels was noticed before PTX, but phosphate levels were diminished at this time, which was not found in some other studies (Malberti, 2010; Martin & González, 2011; Molony & Stephens, 2011). There has been lack of consensus about augmented phosphate concentration in these patients. (Gal-Moscovici & Sprague, 2007). Gardham et al. (2010) found higher intraindividual variation of phosphate in HD patients than in healthy persons. Young et al (2005) also reported that serum phosphate below 3.5 mg/dL was found in patients with low serum albumin concentration, in older age, and whilst using dialysate with higher calcium. It should be mentioned that mineral metabolism in renal failure is deeply connected with many other disease processes, and phosphate concentration changes are only part of multifaceted process of the chronic renal disease. That is why the effect of PTX on bone mineral density in HD patients with secondary HPT depends on pre- and postoperative determination of parathyroid hormone level for prediction of bone health and supplementation of minerals and active vitamin D metabolites after PTX (Cozzolino et al., 2004; Yano et al, 2003).

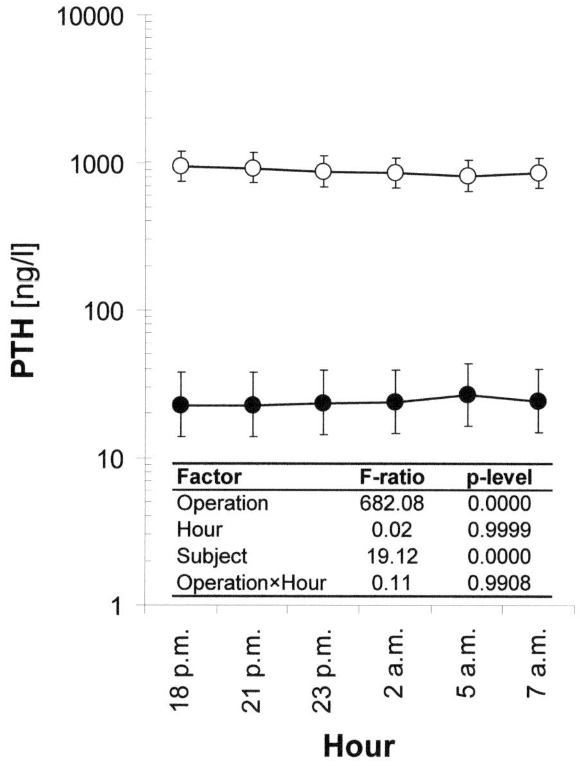

Fig. 2. Nocturnal profiles of parathyroid hormone (PTH) in hemodialyzed patients before and after parathyroidectomy. The drawings and symbols are the same as in Figure 1.

Calcium serum levels were significantly higher before PTX than 1 - 3 months after the operation (Table 1). In HD patients elevated calcium levels are usual (as the reported ones), but not in all cases as published by other authors (Miller et al., 2010). Moreover, abnormalities of both hypo- and hypercalcemia are frequent in patients receiving dialysis therapy, according to Morton et al. (2010). Calcium pull (Pirklbauer & Mayer, 2011) exists in three main forms in the body- the physiologically active free or ionized fraction, a protein bound fraction, and a fraction connected to other anions. Approximately 12% of the bound blood calcium is linked to various anions including phosphate (Ferrari et al., 2009). Ionized calcium is most commonly measured; moreover it is the only physiologically active form of calcium (Monfort et al., 2008). Very close correlation between total and ionized calcium was found ($r = 0.842$; $p < 0.001$) by Carney (1992) and a dialysis did not alter this relationship, despite the obvious significant increase in pH. During dialysis, the ionized calcium fraction decreased and the bound calcium increased along with blood pH. The results of Gosling et al. (1975) however, showed that the fall in ionized calcium and rise in protein-bound calcium are higher and could not be explained only by the redistribution of calcium fractions due to the pH change. At present time, calcium concentration could easily be computed by correcting formulas, obtaining a value of calcium that might possess a significant difference in relation to total calcium. Thus, corrections should be abandoned and preferably ionized calcium should be measured in hemodialysis patients.

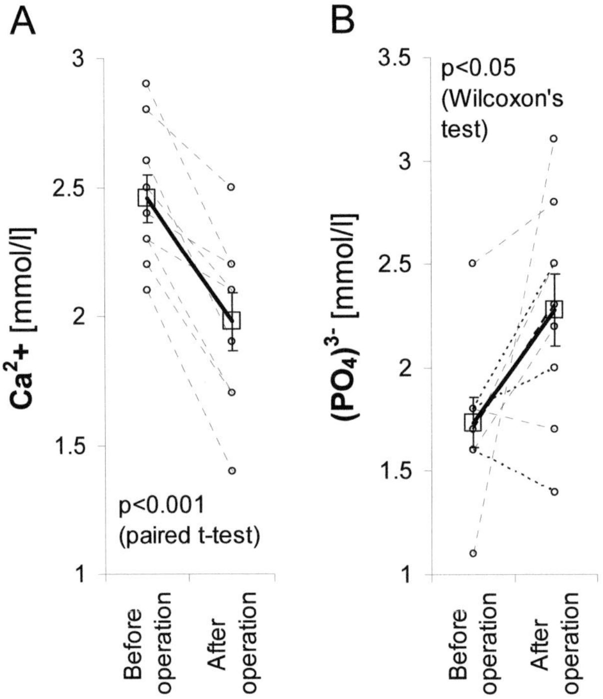

Fig. 3. Changes in serum levels of calcium (section A) and phosphate (section B) after parathyroidectomy. Circles represent experimental points while the squares with error bars represent means ± SEM.

Hypercalcemia, on the other hand, can be associated with increased extraosseous calcium. In general, secretion of parathyroid hormone increases when calcium concentration decreases and vice versa declines when calcium amount rises. Calcitonin also takes part in the regulation of the calcium homeostasis by restraining the bone resorptive effects of parathyroid hormone and also gonadal steroid hormones which enhance the renal and intestinal absorption of calcium. In HD patients with HPT, before PTX, as expected the levels of parathyroid hormone and calcium were high in our study. Parathyroid hormone takes a central role in bone metabolism and bone health. High and low parathyroid hormone levels are connected with high and low turnover bone disease, but high and low parathyroid hormone concentrations are also significantly dependant on age, gender, race, period of hemodialysis and other treatments as well as comorbid conditions (especially

Substance	Before operation						After operation						Diffrerence (After - before operation)					
	n	mean	SD	median	lower quartile	upper quartile	n	mean	SD	median	lower quartile	upper quartile	n	mean	SD	median	lower quartile	upper quartile
PTH [ng/l]	9	1187	626	1373	1089	1683	9	33,73	28,75	38	10	52	9	-1154	631,1	-1361	-1631	-1043
Melatonin [ng/l]	9	29,17	27,33	24,8	10,6	34	9	53,19	40,71	37,2	25	78,5	9	24,02	28,82	13,9	3,4	38
Ca^{2+} [mmol/l]	9	2,456	0,27	2,4	2,3	2,6	9	1,978	0,335	2,1	1,7	2,2	9	-0,48	0,211	-0,5	-0,7	-0,3
PO_4^{2-} [mmol/l]	9	1,733	0,361	1,7	1,6	1,8	9	2,278	0,529	2,3	2	2,5	9	0,544	0,648	0,6	0,2	0,7

* Wilcoxon paired robust test

Table 1. Values of the followed parameters before and after operation as well as their differences

diabetes mellitus) (Sawaya et al., 2002; Young et al., 2005), although Cheng et al. (2011) recommend further investigations about the involvement of gender. Secondary and even tertiary HPT are common in chronic kidney disease. Total PTX is one of the treating options of those disorders. After the operation parathyroid hormone decreases precipitously and remains stable for certain time bellow the normal concentration. Hyperparathyroidism aggravates and complicates chronic kidney disease and the disturbances in mineral metabolism which include not only abnormal mineral metabolism, but also altered bone structure and dangerous extra skeletal calcifications.

It should be mentioned that melatonin influences bone metabolism and possible mechanism/s might involve regulation of parathyroid, calciotropic and gonadal hormones. Long term melatonin administration is rather inhibitory on parathyroid function and bone metabolism.

In spite of the fact that hormonal disturbances are known occurrences in patients with end-stage renal disease (Viljoen et al., 1992), investigation on the function of melatonin have not yielded much information about the relationships between this hormone and parathyroid hormone, bone and kidneys in health, and particularly, in disease. Little is known about melatonin levels in patients with chronic renal failure and HPT. During the diurnal light phase, melatonin levels are very low, i.e. approximately on the baseline level. Changes in usually high nocturnal melatonin concentrations are only with significant meaning. As mentioned above, the PTX in our study resulted in significant increase of nocturnal melatonin in all HD patients, which persisted one to three months after the operation-Figure 1.

Initially, the relation between pineal gland and parathyroid glands was proved by Au & Raisz (1965), Krstic (1966) and also by an application of isotopes (Kiss and al., 1969). It has been found that extirpation of the pineal gland or applying its extracts leads to changes in the morphology of parathyroid glands and in the processes being under their control. The influence of the pineal gland on the parathyroids is a positive one and pinealectomy is inhibitory to parathyroid function. Thus, the pineal gland must be assumed to have a role in the regulation of metabolism and of electrolyte equilibrium (Kiss et al., 1969). Chan et al. (1991) proved that serum calcium levels of hamsters treated with melatonin were significantly low than those in controls. On the other hand, Shoumura et al. (1992) incubated parathyroid glands with melatonin and described that the ultrastructure and secretory activity of the parathyroid glands were affected, but in opposite direction. A decrease was noticed in the functional activity of the glands 1 hour after the treatment. The parathyroid gland cells showed a few pro-secretory granules in the Golgi area, numerous lipid droplets, decrease of the Golgi complex and the cisternae of the rough endoplasmic reticulum. These changes were considered to be suppressive of the synthesis of parathyroid hormone as a result of melatonin action.

Regarding the studies performed in HD patients: Most of them are conducted during the daytime, and the results about melatonin concentration are conflicting. Luedemann et al. (2001) reported that melatonin levels not only before, but also after hemodialysis in HD patients were highly elevated, when compared with melatonin levels of control subjects. On the contrary, Karasek et al. (2002, 2005) discovered diminished melatonin levels in patients with chronic renal disease undergoing hemodialysis in comparison with the ones in healthy controls. One of the possible explanations, according to the authors, is that the decline in melatonin levels is due to impairment in adrenergic function. A further factor which might influence melatonin concentration is the parathyroid hormone. Results concerning the effect of PTX and its impact on melatonin are also inconsistent. Abdel-Wanis et al. (2001) first described a case of coexisting neurofibromatosis, primary HPT due to parathyroid adenoma and osteomalacia. The authors also described a drop in melatonin levels after PTX. On the other hand, Chou et al. (2005) investigating the levels of melatonin after PTX in a patient found no changes in nocturnal melatonin concentration one week after PTX. The result of our study (Kancheva et al., 2008) established increased nocturnal levels in HD patients one to three months after PTX. The existing data also suggest that the pineal gland might be involved in the regulation of calcium metabolism (Carman et al., 1976; Csaba & Barath, 1974; Kiss et al., 1969). Pinealectomy results in decrease in parathyroid glands activity, but the changes are reversed after administration of melatonin.

The effect of melatonin on calcium metabolism might be mediated via parathyroid glands. To asses the effect of pinealectomy, melatonin administration and the influence of lighting conditions Ostrowska et al. (2001; 2003a, 2003b) traced the daily rhythm of selected bone markers in rats. The authors evaluated the levels of serum alkaline phosphatase, carboxyterminal propeptide of type I procollagen as well as cross-linked carboxyterminal telopeptide of type I collagen. Exposure to long days (23.5 h light, 0.5 h dark) was found to be inhibitory on these markers, while short days (23.5 h, dark, 0.5 h light) had a stimulatory effect, proving that lighting condition and melatonin influenced the bone metabolism in rats. Mammalian bone is remodeling continuously by resorption of old bone by osteoclasts and formation of new bone by osteoblasts. Not only melatonin but estradiol, growth factors and cytokines also promote bone formation and might have preventing effect on bone loss (Roth and al., 1999; Wolden-Hanson et al., 2000; Manolagas, 2000; Ladizesky et al., 2003). Osteoblasts also synthesize other proteins which are incorporated into the bone matrix, including osteocalcin and osteonectin. In the same time osteoclasts generate high levels of superoxide anions during bone resorption that take part in the degradative process (Fraser et al., 1996; Melhus et al., 1999; Berger et al., 1999). Melatonin is known as a powerful free-radical scavenger, antioxidant and with its ability to neutralize free radicals. The hormone could stimulate the activity of antioxidative enzymes like superoxide dismutase (Collin-Osdoby et al., 1998; Reiter et al., 2001, 2009).

According to Vaziri et al. (1993) serum melatonin in patients with HD decreases during dialysis with approximately 25%. It was suggested that hypercalcemia itself provokes the increase of melatonin. In volunteers Wikner et al. (1997) proved that indeed exogenous hypercalcaemia influenced melatonin, increased its secretion and serum level by 20% but left urinary melatonin excretion unaffected.

Melatonin is synthesized in bone marrow. Evidences for synthesis in mouse and human bone marrow cells were presented by Tan et al. (1999) and Conti et al (2000). These cells contain aryl-alkyl-N-acetyltransferase activity and express the mRNA encoding hydroxyindole-O-methyltransferase, proving their ability to synthesize melatonin *de novo*. High melatonin levels might have a protective role against oxidative damage in the proliferating hematopoietic cells or in taking part of bone development through osteoblast formation.

The early differentiation and higher expression of bone marker proteins and also the osteogenic differentiation on bone marrow stem cells are evoked by melatonin presence

(Zaminy et al., 2008). Ostrowska et al. (2003b) found a correlation between the higher melatonin levels and low levels of bone forming markers and increased ones of bone resorption markers after pinealectomy in rats. Activities of the osteoblasts and osteoclasts, cultured together with the presence of melatonin, were both diminished judging by specific bone markers of each cell type (Suzuki & Hattori, 2002). The physiological meaning of this fact should be studied considering eventual existing cell-to-cell communications.

The osteoclast activity is regulated by osteoblast produced factors. Some of the factors are matter of current interest and they are: osteoprotegerin (OPG), receptor activator of nuclear factor (NF) –κB (RANK) and RANK ligand (RANKL). It is known that RANKL polypeptide is a type II transmembrane protein and by its expression by osteobalsts it coordinates the bone remodeling by stimulation of bone resorption (which is done by the osteoclasts). Osteoprotegerin is also produced by the osteoblasts and the overexpression of OPG osteoclast production. In brief, the expression of RANKL and OPG decreases coordinates the bone resorption and density positively and negatively, respectively by controlling the activation state of RANK on osteoclasts (Boyle et al, 2003).

Regarding the effect of melatonin on the bone metabolism (Koyama et al., 2002) proved that melatonin at pharmacologic doses increases bone mass by suppressing resorption through down-regulation of RANKL-mediated osteoclast formation and activation.

Recent studies indicated that melatonin may influence bone directly acting on osteoclasts and osteoblasts and/or by down-regulating receptor activator of nuclear factor- κB ligand (RANKL) (Ostrowska et al, 2010).

3. Hyperparathyroidism, parathyroid hormone and steroids in mineral and bone metabolism

The contribution of sex steroids, mainly testosterone and estradiol to bone regulation implies that their dysfunction may be implicated in the emergence of renal osteodystrophy accompanied with HPT in HD men. In male HD patients, the testosterone concentration declined significantly with aging, whereas the esrogen values increased with longer duration of HD. It is generally accepted that estrogens play greater role in maintenance of bone's health than androgens. Testosterone has underlined anti-osteoporotic and beneficial effect on bone metabolism, bone mineral density and maintaining bone mass in men, via direct interaction with androgen receptors. Its influence in the same time is believed to be mediated by estrogen receptors after aromatization of testosterone to bioavailable estradiol.

In postmenopausal women parathyroid hormone suppression by exogenous calcium is reduced. It was suggested that actually estrogen replacement therapy stimulates the parathyroid glands and consequently augments basal parathyroid hormone secretion. To test whether this relationship might be caused by estrogen deficiency 9 postmenopausal women were given transdermal estradiol treatment for 3 months at a dose of 100 μg/day. Parathyroid hormone reactivity to intravenous administration of $CaCl_2$ (10 % solution, 0.2 mL/kg for 5 minutes) was determined before and at the end of the treatment period. Compliance to treatment was evaluated by determination of serum levels of estradiol and FSH. Estradiol was measured by means of an own radioimmunological method (Hampl et al., 1988) and FSH using commercial kit (Kosice, Slovak Republic). Comparing estradiol and FSH values and decremental area of parathyroid hormone and incremental area of calcium before and after estrogen treatment, Student's paired t-test was used. Decremental area of parathyroid hormone and incremental area of calcium were defined as areas circumscribed by baseline and serum levels of these indicators. To see whether the decremental or incremental areas differed significantly from zero Student's one sample t-test was used. The results were then evaluated independently also by a substantially more robust non-statistical, so-called Gnostic method, suited for evaluation of small groups data samples (Baran, 1988; Kovanic, 1986).

Estrogen treatment raised the basal serum estradiol (Zofkova et al. 1993), reduced the corresponding FSH, but left serum calcium and parathyroid hormone levels unchanged as shown in Table 2 and Figure 4.

	Before E_2 treatment	At the end of E_2 treatment	Normal range: Follicular phase	Normal range: Luteal phase	Normal range: Midcycle phase	Normal range: Postmenopausal phase
S-Estradiol (nmol/l)	0.1±0.02	0.46±0.10	0.099-0.95	0.2-1.5	-	0.015-0.160
	$p<0.01$					
S-FSH (U/l)	77.5±7.4	33.9±5.7	2-10	0.5-10	10-30	15-140
	$p<0.001$					
Ca_u mmol/12 h (08:00 - 20:00 h)	5.2±0.4	4.3±0.6	-	-	-	-
Ca_u mmol/12 h (20:00 - 08:00 h)	3.4±0.4	2.7±0.3	-	-	-	-
Ca/Cr index	0.15±0.03	0.10±0.01	normal range up to 0.2			

Results are expressed as mean±SE; n=9.

Table 2. Effect of Estraderm (E2) on serum levels of estradiol and FSH, and urinary excretion of calcium during two 12-h periods following immediately upon an iv calcium load.

Similar urinary calcium excretion values were recorded before and after estradiol treatment (Table 2). Intravenous infusion of $CaCl_2$ induced hypercalcemia as demonstrated in Figure 4.

From Figures 5 and 6 it is apparent that it might be possible to expect that estradiol increases the suppressability of parathyroid hormone (i.e. the ratio of the decremental area of parathyroid hormone after/before >1) in more than 75.8 % and reduces the serum calcium level achieved after a calcium load (i.e. the ratio of the incremental area of calcium after/before <1) in more than 82.1 % of the population of post-menopausal women.

From the results presented it is reasonable to assume that estrogen deficiency contributes to the impaired parathyroid hormone suppressibility. The effect of estradiol on basal hypercalcemia described by other authors (Boucher et al., 1989; Gallagher & Nordin, 1975) was not confirmed. Lower increment of calcemia after estrogen treatment attained by administration of the same calcium load as in the control test does not exclude the possibility that estrogen alters body distribution of calcium.

Renal osteodystrophy is a term used to describe secondary HPT, disorders of bone turnover, abnormalities of calcium and phosphate metabolism, and osteomalacia (Isaia et al., 2008). According to Danese et al. (2006) there are no associations between calcium and phosphate concentrations with the risk of fractures, there are weak with parathyroid hormone, and prospective studies are needed to determine whether therapies that maintain parathyroid hormone concentrations within or near the reasonable range will result in complications of disordered mineral metabolism. Secondary HPT is one of the major abnormalities determining chronic kidney disease as parathyroid hyperplasia very frequently is a result of changed calcium and phosphate metabolism. Fukagawa et al. (2011) consider that mortality rate for patients on HD with secondary HPT is extremely high, many of them are on HD therapy for a longer time and this could increase the prevalence and degree of secondary HPT. In the same time the increase in serum calcium and phosphate that does accompany HPT play a more crucial role in the development of vascular calcification, than HPT itself (Goodman, 2002; Qunibi, 2007; Raggi et al., 2004).

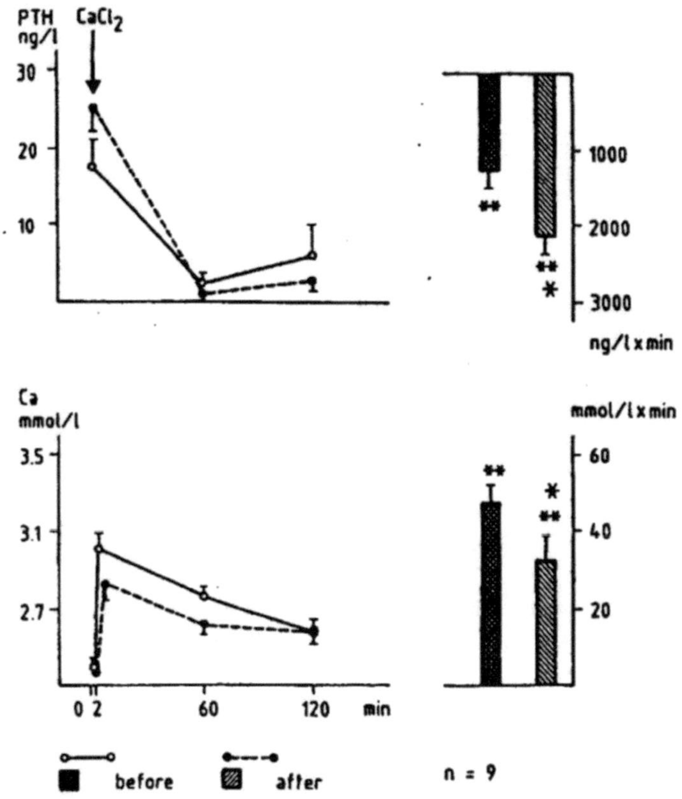

Fig. 4. Serum PTH and calcium responses to iv injection of calcium chloride in 9 postmenopausal women investigated before and after 3 months period of transdermal estradiol treatment. Values denoted are means ± SE (evaluated by paired t test). Normal basic ranges for the various parameters were as follows: serum PTH : 10 - 55 ng/L; total serum calcium: 2.24 - 2.60 nmol/L.

Estrogens could inhibit parathyroid hormone activated bone resorption both *in vitro* and *in vivo*. Estrogens could block parathyroid hormone activated osteoclast formation by abolishing parathyroid hormone responsive cyclic adenosine monophosphate (cAMP) pathway in mouse bone culture (Kaji et al., 1996; Kanatani et al., 1998). It was determined that estrogen inhibits parathyroid hormone-stimulated osteoclast formation by directly acting on hemopoietic blast cells in mouse and rat, possibly through blocking the cAMP-dependent protein kinase pathway but not the calcium/protein kinase C pathway (Kanatani et al., 1998).

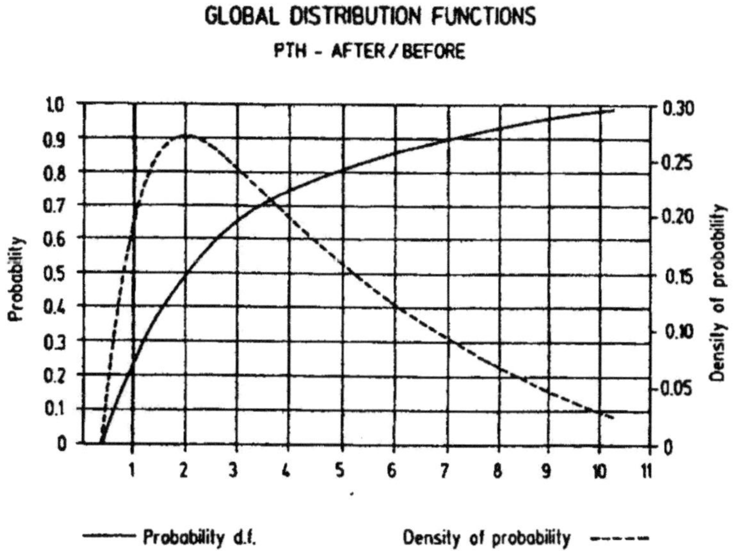

Fig. 5. Global distribution function and density of the decremental PTH area ratio after/before E2 (evaluated by gnostical method). It appears that the sample of ratio can be considered as homogenous. The probability of a ratio not to exceed 1 (the risk of negative result of the treatment) is estimated as 0.242 for the original data.

More recent findings related to the putative role of fibroblast growth factor 23 (FGF-23) on the estrogen receptors support the conception of indirect effects of estrogens on bone metabolism and on the regulation of parathyroid hormone by estrogens. It is likely that FGF-23 mediates its functions through FGF receptors (FGFR1) and the co-receptor Klotho. In addition, FGF23 has ability to reduce parathyroid hormone secretion (Jüppner et al., 2010; Nakai et al., 2010). However, during the early stages of chronic kidney disease, increased FGF-23 production enhances phosphate excretion, prevents the development of hyperphosphatemia, reduces the circulating levels of $1,25(OH)_2$ vitamin D_3, and subsequently contributes to the development of secondary HPT. In patients undergoing HD, FGF-23 levels are elevated in response to hyperphosphatemia and eventually to vitamin D therapy, but fail to suppress the secretion of parathyroid hormone. Experimental data suggests that the parathyroid resistance to FGF-23 may be caused by decreased expression of Klotho-FGFR1 complex in hyperplastic parathyroid glands (Komaba & Fukagawa, 2010).

Estrogens are supposed to have both direct and indirect effects on bone via the estrogen receptor α and estrogen receptor β. They exert estrogen-dependent parathyroid hormone suppression but the mechanisms by which estrogens modulate parathyroid hormone are controversial. Carrillo-López et al. (2009) investigated the levels of parathyroid hormone in a combined rat model (i.e. rats with chronic kidney disease and ovariectomy). Estrogens were administered to the animals and the authors proved that the estrogen treatment significantly decreased both parathyroid hormone mRNA and serum levels as well, but did not find any estrogen receptor α or β mRNA or protein in the parathyroid glands. These results pointed out an indirect effect of estrogen action on parathyroid hormone regulation. In the same time estrogen treatment significantly decreased serum $1{,}25(OH)_2$ vitamin D_3 and phosphate concentrations. Fibroblast growth factor 23 mRNA levels were increased as a result of the estrogen treatment. Experiments *in vitro* shown that estrogens led to up-regulation of FGF23 in osteoblast-like cells in a time- and dose-dependent manner, suggesting that parathyroid hormone is regulated indirectly by estrogens, probably trough FGF-23.

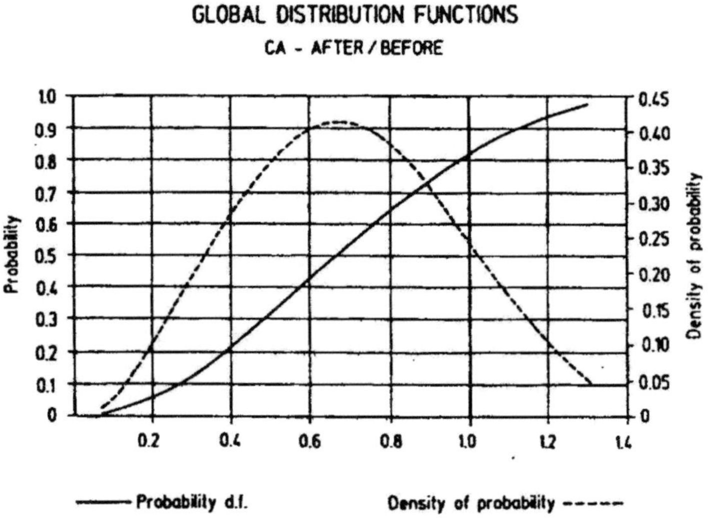

Fig. 6. Global distribution function and density of the incremental calcium area ratio after/before before E2 (evaluated by gnostical method). The probability of failing treatment (of a ratio exceeding 1) is 0.179 for the original data.

The recent experiments outline that estrogens suppress parathyroid hormone synthesis and secretion in concentration-dependent manner, probably mainly by an indirect mechanism. Additionally, the calcium-phosphate-vitamin D-parathyroid hormone axis can also be indirectly affected by estrogens (Cannata-Andía et al., 2010). In addition, fibroblast growth factor 23 also positively correlates with the concentration of estrogens.

Androgens are also supposed to regulate bone metabolism in mammals. Testosterone inhibits osteoclast formation by parathyroid hormone, but through an androgen receptor. Gonadal androgen steroids act also directly on osteoblasts by binding to androgen receptors. Chen et al. (2001) performed a study to investigate if testosterone and DHT would influence osteoclast formation stimulated by parathyroid hormone and $1{,}25(OH)_2$ vitamin D_3 in mouse bone cell culture. Induced osteoclast formation was inhibited in concentration-dependently manner by testosterone and even stronger by DHT, but the one activated by $1{,}25(OH)_2$ vitamin D_3 was not blocked. Applying in their experiment a specific estrogen antagonist and an aromatase inhibitor the authors confirmed that testosterone inhibited osteoclast formation induced by parathyroid hormone through the androgen receptor, but not through the production of estrogen by aromatization of androgen.

In bone tissue both androgen and estrogen receptor are expressed. Wiren et al (2008) used transgenic mice population with overexpressed androgen receptors. The authors found that enhanced androgen signaling results in low bone turnover and inhibition of bone formation by differentiated osteoblasts and that androgen action on mature osteoblast is not anabolic.

Anabolic steroids have been applied to treat patients with osteoporosis. They might act directly on the bone tissue, but it has been also suggested that they have an indirect effect, exerted via changes in the secretion of calcitonin (Salamano et al., 1990). Moreover, a positive correlation between the levels of testosterone and calcitonin has recently been found (Liu et al., 2011). A direct relationship between parathyroid hormone and androgens is not elucidated. In order to test the effect of synthetic anabolic steroid (synthetic androgen) on calcium- induced suppressibility of parathyroid hormone in postmenopausal women stanazolol (Stromba®, Sterling products, UK) was orally given for 1 month in daily dose of 10 mg to postmenopausal women with osteoporosis. Each woman had two identical i.v. $CaCl_2$ tests (10 % CaCl2, at a dose of 0.2 mL/kg body weight for 5 minutes) - one before and the other at the end of the treatment period. Serum parathyroid hormone, LH, testosterone, and ionized calcium were determined in blood samples taken before, 5, 60 and 120 minutes after the calcium loading. Student's paired t-test was used when the decremental parathyroid hormone and the incremental calcium areas were compared before and after the stanazolol treatment. The same test was also used when comparing basal values for the various parameters before and after the treatment.

Exogenous hypercalcemia suppressed serum parathyroid hormone almost identically before and after stanazolol treatment, as reflected by the decremental areas of parathyroid hormone (Figure 7). The calcium induced hypercalcemia expressed as an incremental area of calcium was of a similar magnitude before and after the drug application (Figure 7).

Stanazolol reduced the serum LH from 38 ±4 to 30 ± 3 UI/L ($p < 0.01$) and testosterone from 0.77 ± 0.10 to 0.44 ± 0.08 nmol/L ($p < 0.05$), which confirmed that a good compliance was achieved by the treatment. In conclusion, the study does not support the hypothesis that the effect of stanazolol on bone is mediated by an alteration of parathyroid hormone secretion (Zofkova et al, 1994).

The androgen receptor mediates biological responses to androgens (Clarke & Khosia, 2009). Since androgens can be converted into estrogen, the specific role of the androgen receptors in mineral metabolism and homeostasis remains controversial. Kenny et al. (1998) found that in old age testosterone concentrations were below the normal range in 38 % of men, and parathyroid hormone levels were elevated in 23 of them, but there is no other data available about the direct relationship between these two hormones.

4. Hyperparathyroidism and gonadotropic hormones

Reproductive hormone concentrations are influenced in chronic renal failure. With the progression of the kidney disease (and with the introduction of systematic HD) sexual and gonadotropic hormone concentrations are affected. Decrease in plasma testosterone and

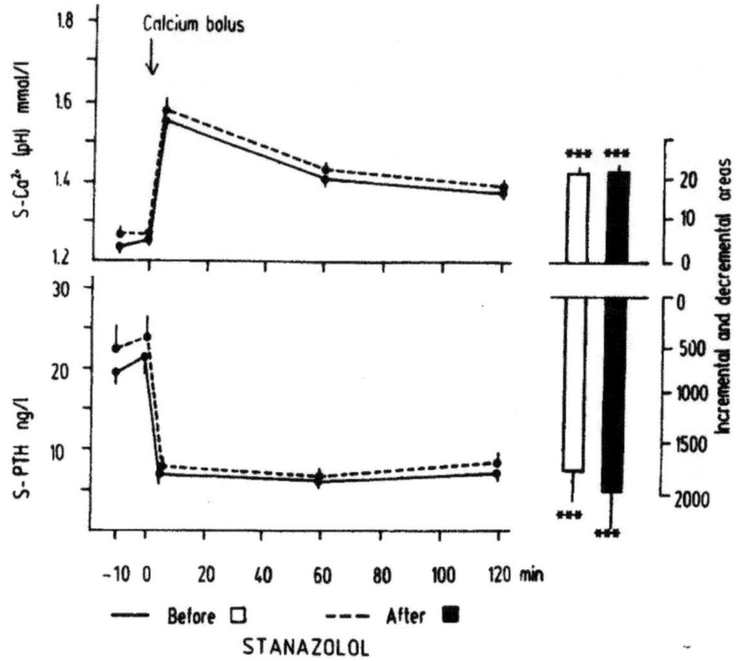

Fig. 7. Left panel. Serum ionized calcium (corrected by pH - Ca $^{2+}$ /pH) and PTH response to iv calcium before after 1 month's treatment with stanazolol in 11 postmenopusal women. Values denoted are means ± SEM. Normal basal range for serum ionized calcium are 1.17 - 1.29 mmol/L and PTH 12 - 55 ng/L. Right panel. Corresponding incremental and decremental areas.

estradiol also affect bone metabolism and bone mineral density. Impotence and azoospermia are usual among male patients undergoing a chronic HD program. The current evidence suggests that androgens have direct beneficial effects on bone metabolism. Follicle stimulating hormone (FSH) and luteinizing hormone (LH) are suspected to be negatively associated with bone mineral status. The relative contribution and relationships among testosterone, LH, FSH and parathyroid hormone in HD patients with HPT are still not well known and deserve elucidation.

The function of the adenohypophyseal-gonadal axis in HD male patients is modified: the serum testosterone concentration is low, and the gonadotropin levels are increased. The pathogenetic role of secondary HPT in this disorder seems not to be fully defined. The effect of secondary hyperparathyroidism upon hormones of the pituitary-testicular axis was studied by Bogićević & Stefanović (1988) in end-stage kidney disease male patients on maintenance HD. A significant positive correlation was found between the serum levels of PTH and LH (r = 0.405). Akmal et al. (1988) described an important role for the excess blood levels of PTH in uremia in the genesis of the hypotestosteronemia.

To test the effect of PTX on the secretion of LH, FSH, and testosterone seven HD men with advanced secondary HPT (in whom PTX was performed) were included in the study. Nine healthy men served as controls. Three identical gonadotropin releasing hormone (GnRH) tests (0.1 mg over a period of 30 seconds) were performed for each patient - before PTX, 3 and 6 months after the operation and one for the controls. Blood samples for the determination of serum LH, FSH, and testosterone were taken before (time 0) and 20, 40, 60, 80, and 100 minutes after the treatment with GnRH. Serum intact parathyroid hormone, $1{,}25(OH)_2$ vitamin D_3, 25(OH) vitamin D_3, total calcium, phosphate, prolactin, hemoglobin, and hematocrit were estimated at time 0. Decremental areas under the curve (AUC) for LH, FSH, and testosterone were determined. The AUC is defined as an area circumscribed by the joint line of values measured at 0, 20, 40, 60, 80, and 100 minutes after the GnRH administration and the horizontal line provided by the values at time 0. Bonferroni test was used to compare the AUC values of LH, FSH, and testosterone as well as through the second period after the PTX.

Serum parathyroid hormone, calcium, and phosphate prior to PTX markedly exceeded the upper limit of reference values. These indices decreased in all of the investigated patients at the third month after the operation ($p<0.01$, $p<0.01$ and $p<0.1$, respectively, as compared with the mean values before the operation – Table 3).

	Normal range	Before PTX	After PTX	
			3rd month	6th month
Serum intact PTH, ng/l	10. 0 - 65	956. 1 ± 115.7	81.0 ± 34.0 [a]	138.1 ± 57.1 [a]
Total calcium, mmol/l	2. 20 - 2. 60	2.44 ± 0.04	2.11 ± 0.09 [a]	2.23 ± 0.13 [a]
Phosphates, mmol/l	0. 80 - 1.62	2.25 ± 0.09	1.55 ± 0.08 [a]	1.78 ± 0.12 [a]
$1.25(OH)_2D_3$, ng/l	18.0 - 62. 0	14.44 ± 4.41	37.81 ± 7.57 [b]	27. 6 ± 1. 17 [b]
$25(OH)D_3$, ng/ml	16.0 - 74. 0	11.72 ± 1. 35	18. 91 ± 2.47	18.91 ± 4. ±
Prolaktin, µg/l	3.0 - 17.7	43.23 ± 17.21	47. 79 ± 18.87	41.54 ± 15.92
Haemoglobin, g/l		81.2 ± 7.66	87. 2 ± 5.78	25. 8 ± 2.1
Haematocrit, %				

The Bonferroni test was calculated for n = 7.
[a] $p<0.01$ as compared with the values before PTX.
[b] $p<0.05$ as compared with the values before PTX. There were no differences between those values of the first and the second postoperative in any of the investigated parameters

Table 3. Serum intact PTH, total calcium, phosphates, $1{,}25\ (OH)_2D_3$, 25(OH) vitamin D_3, prolactin, haemoglobin, haematocrit in dialyzed men before and 3 and 6 months after PTX (mean ± SEM)

At the sixth month, the mean serum parathyroid hormone and phosphate levels were lower ($p<0.01$ and $p<0.05$ as compared with the same values before PTX) although an increasing tendency in both parameters was apparent. However, the changes of these concentrations were not significant when compared with the values at the third month (Table 3).

Serum $1{,}25(OH)_2$ vitamin D_3 increased in all except one patients after three months ($p<0.01$, table 1), and sixth months after PTX ($p<0.01$ as compared with the concentration before PTX, Table 3). The response of serum 25(OH) vitamin D_3 to PTX was not as significant early after PTX as later (Table 3). In HD patients serum testosterone concentrations were lower as compared in healthy men, and the secretory response to GnRH was very flat. The peaks in testosterone secretion recorded in the healthy subjects at the 40th and 100th min after GnRH applications were not observed either before or after PTX. There were no differences between the mean concentrations of basal or GnRH-induced testosterone AUC levels either before PTX or during both periods after the operation (Figure 8). The basal serum LH

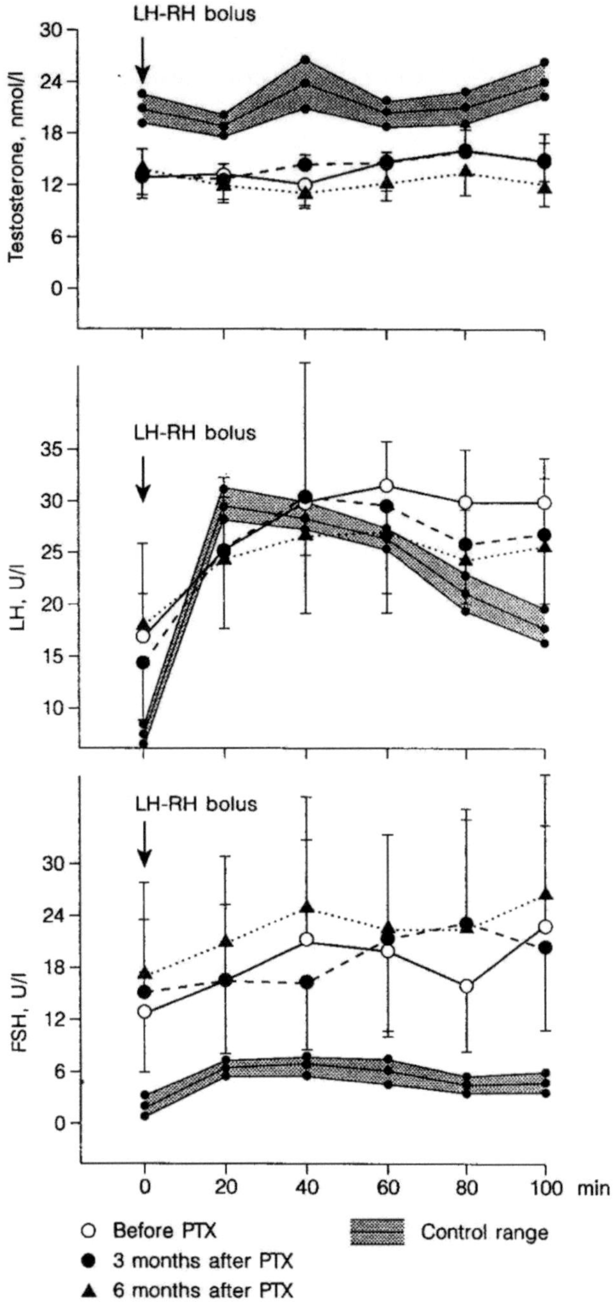

Fig. 8. Testosterone, LH and FSH responses to LH-RH before PTX (open circles and soild lines), at 3rd month after PTX (closed circules, and dashed lines), and at 6th month after PTH (triangles and dotted lines). The values are means ± SEM, evaluated by Bonferroni test for n = 7. The shaded area represents the mean values ± SEM of 9 healthy men (mean age 29.8, range 20 - 38 years) who did not take any form of medication.

concentrations exceeded the upper limit of the normal male range. The AUC was 1.110 ± 223 UI/L x min. The secretion kinetics of the gonadotropic hormone after GnRH administration was altered in the patients before and during the first and second periods after PTX, the increase being slower so that the peak is reached later as compared with healthy men (between the 40th and the 60th min after GnRH stimulation). Thereafter, a plateau followed instead of a decline as registered in the case of healthy men. No significant differences between LH AUC values before or after the PTX were observed.

The serum concentrations of FSH were higher in HD patients before and after PTH as compared with healthy subjects. The secretion kinetics of FSH before and after PTH was very similar. Serum prolactin exceeded the upper range of normal values and before and also after the PTX. No correlations were observed between parathyroid hormone, calcium, phosphate, 1,25(OH)$_2$ vitamin D$_3$, or 25(OH) vitamin D$_3$ and AUC values of testosterone, LH, FSH, prolactin either before PTX or after the operation. Taken as a whole, the obtained data show that adenohypophyseal-gonadal dysfunction in HD men is not dependent on the activity of the parathyroid hormone-1,25(OH)$_2$ vitamin D$_3$ axis (Zofkova et al., 1996). Fujii et al. (1986) have found a long lasting alteration in the hypothalamo-pituitary- gonadal axis in the female offspring rats born to PTX mothers. The authors observed a decrease in GnRH-stimulated release of LH and FSH in the PTX first generation rats, more pronounced in females at 14 and 22 days of age. An association of increased parathyroid hormone and decreased vitamin D metabolite was detected in patients obesity by Panidis et al. (2005), but they did not report any existing relation between FSH, LH and parathyroid hormone. Inappropriately low concentrations of FSH and LH with respect to sex steroids were measured by Rochira et al. (2007) in a subject with osteopenia and aromatase deficiency, but also no other relations between the hormones were described. Castelo-Branco et al. (2008) evaluated the effect of FSH levels in the development of human osteoporosis and found that bone mineral density correlated positively with the FSH levels, but did not appear to have a major role in the development of bone loss in young women with primary amenorrhea. The authors also did not announce any relationships between parathyroid hormone concentrations and FSH.

5. Concluding remarks

In hemodialyzed patients with secondary hyperparathyroidism, parathyroidectomy significantly increased the nocturnal secretion of melatonin. The increased parathyroid hormone levels have been related to lower melatonin levels. Removal of the pineal gland or administration of its extracts produces alterations in the morphology and hormonal secretion of the parathyroid glands. Patients with end stage renal disease or on systematic HD suffer from related to melatonin disorders. The pineal gland and melatonin might be assumed as one of the regulating factors of the metabolism and electrolyte equilibrium. Despite some controversial results, data indicates that pineal melatonin is involved in the regulation of calcium and phosphate metabolism by stimulating the activity of the parathyroid glands and by inhibiting calcitonin release. It is supposed that hypercalcemia itself provokes an increase of melatonin and that exogenous hypercalcaemia has impact on melatonin levels, increasing its secretion and serum level by 20%. Osteoclasts generate high levels of superoxide anions during bone resorption that take part in the degradative process. Additionally, melatonin is known as a powerful free-radical scavenger, antioxidant and with its ability to neutralize free radicals, and thus promotes bone formation and prevents bone resorption. Melatonin is synthesized in bone marrow cells. These cells contain aryl-alkyl-N-acetyltransferase activity and express the mRNA encoding hydroxyindole-O-methyltransferase, proving their ability to synthesize melatonin *de novo,* which might have protective role against oxidative damage in the proliferating hematopoietic cells or in taking part of bone development through osteoblast formation. It is suspected that melatonin might affect the bone directly acting on osteoclasts and osteoblasts and by suppressing resorption through down-regulation of RANKL-mediated osteoclast formation and activation.

The contribution of sex steroids to bone regulation implies that their dysfunction may be complicated by renal osteodystrophy accompanied with HPT in HD patients. Testosterone has pronounced anti-osteoporotic and beneficial effect on bone metabolism, bone mineral density and maintaining bone mass in men. Testosterone's effect (at least part of it) is believed to be mediated by estrogen receptors after aromatization of testosterone to bioavailable estradiol. From the results obtained it is possible to assume that estrogen deficiency contributes to the impaired parathyroid hormone suppressibility and alters body distribution of calcium. Increased serum calcium and phosphate along with HPT play more crucial role in the development of vascular calcification, than HPT itself.

Estrogens have direct and indirect effects on bone via the estrogen receptor α and estrogen receptor β. There are evidences that estrogen suppresses parathyroid hormone synthesis and secretion in concentration-dependent manner, probably mainly by an indirect mechanism. The concept of the indirect effect of estrogens on bone metabolism and on the parathyroid hormone regulation recently is supported by the putative role of fibroblast growth factor 23 (FGF-23) and the co-receptor Klotho on the estrogen receptors.

The direct relationship between parathyroid hormone and androgens is not elucidated. The effect of synthetic androgen stanazolol on calcium - induced suppressibility of parathyroid hormone in postmenopausal women does not support the hypothesis that the effect of stanazolol on bone is mediated by alteration of parathyroid hormone secretion.

In chronic renal disease, the levels of gonadal hormones are usually influenced. As kidney disease progresses and with the introduction of systematic HD the sexual and the adenohypophyseal gonadotropic hormones are commonly affected. Pituitary-gonadal axis in HD patients with HPT is also affected and modified, i.e. the serum testosterone concentration is low and gonadotropin levels are increased. No correlations have been found between the parathyroid hormone, LH, FSH, prolactin, calcium, phosphate, $1{,}25(OH)_2$ vitamin D_3 and 25(OH) vitamin D_3 values before or after the performed PTX in our already mentioned study. Probably, adenohypophyseal-gonadal dysfunction in men on HD does not dependent on the activity of the parathyroid hormone-$1{,}25(OH)_2$ vitamin D_3 axis.

6. Acknowledgements

Supported by a grant project NS/9831-4 of the Internal Grant Agency of the Czech Republic.

7. References

Abdel-Wanis, ME., Kawahara, N & Tomita, K. (2001). The association of neurofibromatosis 1 and spinal deformity with primary hyperparathyroidism and osteomalacia might melatonin have a role? *J Orthop Sci* ,Vol. 6, № 2 (Mar 2001), pp. 193-198, ISSN 0949-2658

Akmal, M., Goldstein, DA., Kletzky, OA. & Massry, SG.(1988). Hyperparathyroidism and hypotestosteronemia of acute renal failure. *Am J Nephrol*, Vol. 8, № 2 (Feb 1988), pp. 166-169, ISSN 0250-8095

Allan, CM., Kalak, R., Dunstan, CR., McTavish, KJ., Zhou, H., Handelsman, DJ. & Seibel MJ. (2010). Follicle-stimulating hormone increases bone mass in female mice. *Proc Natl Acad Sci USA*, Vol. 107, №52, (Dec 2010), pp. 2629-2634, ISSN 0027-8424

Ashida, K., Akehi, Y., Kudo, T. & Yanase, T. (2010). Bone and Men's Health. The role of androgens in bone metabolism. *Clin. Calcium*, Vol. 20, № 2 (Feb 2010), pp. 165-173, ISSN 0917 -5857

Au, WY. & Raisz, LG. (1965). Effect of vitamin D and dietary calcium on parathyroid activity. *Am J Physiol*, Vol. 209, № 3, (Sep 1965), pp. 637-662, ISSN 0002-9513

Baran, RH. (1988). Comments on „A new theoretical and algorithmical basis for estimation, identification and control" by P.Kovanic. *Automatica*. Vol. 24, № 2, (1988), pp. 283-287, ISSN 0005-1098

Berger, CE., Horrocks, BR & Datta, HK. (1999). Direct non-genomic effect of steroid hormones on superoxide anion generation in the bone resorbing osteoclasts. *Mol Cell Endocrinol*, Vol. 149, № 1-2, (Mar 1999), pp. 53-59, ISSN 0303-7207

Block, GA., Klassen, PS., Lazarus, JM., Ofsthun, N., Lowrie, EG. & Chertow, GM. (2004). Mineral metabolism, mortality, and morbidity in maintenance hemodialysis. *J Am Soc Nephrol*, Vol. 15, № 8, (Aug 2004), pp. 2208-2218, ISSN 1046-6673

Bogićević, M. & Stefanović, V. (1988). Relationship between parathyroid hormone and pituitary-testicular axis in patients on maintenance hemodialysis. *Exp Clin Endocrinol*, Vol. 92, № 3, (Mar 1988), pp. 357-362, ISSN 0232-7384

Boyle, WJ., Simonet, WS. & Lacey DL. (2003). Osteoclast differentiation and activation. *Nature*, Vol. 423, № 6937, (May 2003), pp. 337-342, ISSN 0028-0836

Boucher, A., D'Amour, P., Hamel, L., Fugère, P., Gascon-Barré, M., Lepage, R. & Ste-Marie, LG. (1989). Estrogen replacement decreases the set point of parathyroid hormone stimulation by calcium in normal postmenopausal women. *J Clin Endocrinol Metab*, Vol. 68, № 4, (Apr 1989), pp. 831-836, ISSN 0021-972X

Cannata-Andía, JB., Carrillo-López, N. & Naves-Díaz, M. (2010) Estrogens and bone disease in chronic kidney disease role of FGF23. *Curr Opin Nephrol Hypertens*, Vol. 19, № 4 (Jul 2010), pp. 354-358, ISSN 1062-4821

Cardinali, DP., Ladizesky, MG., Boggio, V., Cutrera, RA. & Mautalen, C. (2003). Melatonin effects on bone experimental facts and clinical perspectives. *J Pineal Res*, Vol. 34, № 2, (Mar 2003), pp. 81-87, ISSN 0742-3098

Carrillo-López, N., Román-García, P., Rodríguez-Rebollar, A., Fernández-Martín, JL., Naves-Díaz, M. & Cannata-Andía, JB.(2009). Indirect regulation of PTH by estrogens may require FGF23. *Am Soc Nephrol*, Vol. 20, № 9 (Sep 2009) pp. 2009-2017, ISSN 1046-6673

Carman, JS., Post, RM., Buswell, R. & Goodwin, FK. (1976). Negative effects of melatonin on depression. *Am J Psychiatry*, Vol. 133, № 10 (Oct 1976), pp. 1181-1186, ISSN 0002-953X

Carney, SL. (1992). Ionized calcium concentration in maintenance hemodialysis patients. *Clin Nephrol*, Vol. 38, № 3 (Sep 1992), pp. 167-170, ISSN 0301-0430.

Castelo-Branco, C., León, M., Durán, M., & Balasch J. (2008). Follicle-stimulating hormone does not directly regulate bone mass in human beings evidence from nature. *Fertil Steril*, Vol. 90, № 6, (Dec 2008), pp. 2211-2216, ISSN 0015-0282

Chan, H., Shoumura, S., Emura, S., Utsumi, M., Yamahira, T. & Isono, H. (1991). Effect of melatonin on ultrastructure of the golden hamster parathyroid gland. *Histol Histopath.*, Vol. 6, № 1 (Jan 1991), pp. 1-7, ISSN 0213-3911

Chan, HW., Chu, KH., Fung, SK., Tang, HL., Lee, W., Cheuk, A., Yim, KF., Tong, MK. & Lee, KC. (2010a) Prospective study on dialysis patients after total parathyroidectomy without autoimplant. *Nephrology* (Carlton), Vol. 15, № 4 (Jun 2010), pp. 441-447, ISSN 1320-5358

Chen, Q., Kaji, H., Sugimoto, T. & Chihara, K. (2001). Testosterone inhibits osteoclast formation stimulated by parathyroid hormone through androgen receptor. *FEBS Lett*, Vol. 491, № 1-2, (Feb 2001), pp. 91-93, ISSN 0014-5793

Cheng, SP., Yang, TL., Lee, JJ., Chen, HH., Wu, CJ., Liu, TP. & Liu, CL. (2011). Gender differences among patients with secondary hyperparathyroidism undergoing parathyroidectomy. *J Surg Res.*, Vol. 168, № 1, (Jun 2011), pp. 82-87, ISSN 0022-4804

Chou, FF., Lee, CH., Chen, JB., Huang, SC. & Lee, CT. (2005). Sleep disturbances before and after parathyroidectomy for secondary hyperparathyroidism. *Surgery*, Vol. 137, № 4, (Apr 2005), pp. 426-430, ISSN 0039-6060

Clarke, BL. & Khosla, S. (2009). Androgens and bone. *Steroids*, Vol. 74, № 3 (Mar 2009), pp. 296-305, ISSN 0039-128X

Collin-Osdoby, P., Li, L., Rothe, L., Anderson, F., Kirsch, D., Oursler, MJ. & Osdoby, P. (1998). Inhibition of avian osteoclast bone resorption by monoclonal antibody 121F a mechanism involving the osteoclast free radical system. *J Bone Miner Res*,Vol. 13, № 1, (Jan 1998), pp. 67-78, ISSN 0884-0431

Conti, A., Conconi, S., Hertens, E., Skwarlo-Sonta, K., Markowska, M. & Maestroni, JM. (2000). Evidence for melatonin synthesis in mouse and human bone marrow cells. *J Pineal Res*, Vol. 28, № 4, (May 2000), pp. 193-202, ISSN 0742-3098

Cozzolino, M., Gallieni, M., Corsi, C. & Bastagli, A. Brancaccio, D. (2004). Management of calcium refilling post-parathyroidectomy in end-stage renal disease. *J Nephrol*, Vol. 17, № 1, (Jan-Feb 2004), pp. 3-8, ISSN 1121-8428

Csaba, G. & Barath, P. (1974). The effect of pinealectomy on the parafollicular cells of the rat thyroid gland. *Acta Anat (Basel)*,Vol. 88, № 1, (Jan 1974), pp. 137-146, ISSN 0001-5180

Csaba, G. & Bókay, J. (1977). The effect of melatonin and corpus pineale extract on serum electrolytes in the rat. *Acta Biol Acad Sci Hung.*, Vol. 28, № 1, (Jan 1977), pp. 143-144, ISSN 0001-5288

Danese, MD., Kim, J., Doan, QV., Dylan, M., Griffiths, R. & Chertow, GM. (2006). PTH and the risks for hip, vertebral, and pelvic fractures among patients on dialysis. *Am J Kidney Dis*, Vol. 47, №1, (Jan 2006), pp. 149-156, ISSN 0272-6386

Doumouchtsis, KK., Perrea, DN. & Doumouchtsis, SK. (2009). The impact of sex hormone changes on bone mineral deficit in chronic renal failure. *Endocr Res*, Vol. 34, № 3, (Aug2009), pp. 90-99, ISSN 0743-5800

Doumouchtsis, KK., Kostakis, AI., Doumouchtsi, SK., Grapsa, E., Passalidou, IA., Tziamalis, MP., Poulakou, MV., Vlachos, IS. & Perrea, DN. (2008). The effect of sexual hormone abnormalities on proximal femur bone mineral density in hemodialysis patients and the possible role of RANKL. *Hemodial Int*, Vol. 12, № 1, (Jan 2008), pp. 100-107, ISSN 1492-7535

Ebeling, PR. Androgens and osteoporosis. (2010). *Curr Opin Endocrinol Diabetes Obes*, Vol. 17, №3, (Jun 2010), pp. 284-292, ISSN 1752-296X

Ebeling, PR. (1998). Osteoporosis in men. New insights into aetiology, pathogenesis, prevention and management. *Drugs Aging, Vol.* 13, №6, (Dec 1998), pp. 421-434, ISSN 1170-229X

Ferrari, P., Singer, R., Agarwal, A., Hurn, A., Townsend, MA. & Chubb, P. (2009) Serum phosphate is an important determinant of corrected serum calcium in end-stage kidney disease. *Nephrology (Carlton)*,Vol. 14, № 4, (Jun 2009), pp. 383-388, ISSN 1320-5358

Fraser, JHE., Helfrivh, MH., Wallace, HM. & Ralston, HM. (1996). Hydrogen peroxide, but not superoxide, stimulates bone resorption in mouse calvariae. *Bone,* Vol. 19, № 3, (Sept 1996), pp. 223-226, ISSN 8756-3282

Fraser, S., Cowen, P., Franklin, M., Franer, C. & Arendt, J. (1983). Direct radioimmunoassay for melatonin in plasma. *Clin Chem,* Vol. 29, № 2, (Feb 1983), pp. 396-397, ISSN 0009-9147

Fujii, T., Yamamoto, N. & Hayashi, K. (1986). Effects of parathyroidectomy in pregnant rats on the luteinizing hormone and follicle-stimulating hormone response to synthetic luteinizing hormone-releasing hormone in the infantile offspring. *Exp Clin Endocrinol.*, Vol. 87, № 2, (Jul 1986), pp. 149-156, ISSN 0232-7384

Fukagawa, M., Komaba, H., Onishi, Y., Fukuhara, S., Akizawa, T. & Kurokawa, K. (2011). Mineral Metabolism Management in Hemodialysis Patients with Secondary Hyperparathyroidism in Japan Baseline Data from the MBD-5D. *Am J Nephrol*, Vol. 33, № 5 (May 2011), pp. 427-437, ISSN 0250-8095

Gal-Moscovici, A. & Sprague, SM. (2007). Bone health in chronic kidney disease-mineral and bone disease. *Adv Chronic Kidney Dis*, Vol. 14, № 1, (Jan 2007), pp. 27-36, ISSN 1548-5595

Gardham, C., Stevens, PE., Delaney, MP., LeRoux, M., Coleman, A. & Lamb, EJ. (2010). Variability of parathyroid hormone and other markers of bone mineral metabolism in patients receiving hemodialysis. *Clin J Am Soc Nephrol*, Vol. 5, № 7, (Jul 2010), pp. 1261-1267, ISSN 1555-9041

Gennari, L., Nuti, R.& Bilezikian, JP. (2004) Aromatase activity and bone homeostasis in men. *J Clin Endocrinol Metab*, Vol. 89, № 12, (Dec 2004), pp. 5898-5907, ISSN 0021-972X

Goodman, WG. (2002). Vascular calcification in end-stage renal disease. *J Nephrol*, Vol. 15, (Suppl 6), (Nov-Dec 2002), pp. 82-85, ISSN 1121-8428

Gosling, P., Robinson, BH. & Sammons, HG. (1975). Changes in protein-bound calcium in the serum of haemodialysis patients. *Clin Sci Mol Med*, Vol. 48, № 6, (Jun 1975), pp. 521-528, ISSN 0144-4107

Hamada, Y. & Fukagawa, M. (2009). Chronic kidney disease (CKD) and bone. The mechanisms of chronic kidney disease--mineral and bone disorder (CKD-MBD). *Clin Calcium,* Vol. 19, № 4, (Apr 2009), pp. 486-492, ISSN 0917 -5857

Hampl, R., Zverina, J., Sulcova, J. & Starka, L. (1988) Steroid and steroid regulating hormones in human male castrates. *Exp Clin Endocrinol*, Vol. 92, № 3, (Mar 1988), pp. 257-261, ISSN 0232-7384

Heaton, JP., Morales, A. (2001). Andropause--a multisystem disease. *Can J Urol*, Vol. 8, № 2, (Apr 2001), pp. 1213-1222, ISSN 1195-9479

Hutchison, AJ., Whitehouse, RW., Boulton, HF., Adams, JE., Mawer, EB., Freemont, TJ., Gokal, R. (1993). Correlation of bone histology with parathyroid hormone, vitamin D3, and radiology in end-stage renal disease. *Kidney Int*, Vol. 44, № 5, (Nov 1993), pp. 1071-1077, ISSN 0085-2538

Jüppner, H., Wolf, M., & Salusky, IB. (2010). FGF-23 More than a regulator of renal phosphate handling? *J Bone Miner Res* ,Vol. 25, № 10, (Oct 2010), pp. 2091-2097, ISSN 0884-0431

Isaia, GC., Tamone, C. & Ravazzoli, M. (2008). Fractures and chronic renal insufficiency. *G Ital Nefrol*, Vol. 25, № 1 (Jan-Feb, 2008), pp. 57-65, ISSN 0393-5590

Kaji, H., Sugimoto, T., Kanatani, M., Nasu, M. & Chihara, K. (1996). Estrogen blocks parathyroid hormone (PTH)-stimulated osteoclast-like cell formation by selectively affecting PTH-responsive cyclic adenosine monophosphate pathway. *Endocrinology*, Vol. 137, № 6, (Jun 1996), pp. 2217-2224, ISSN 0013-7227

Kanatani, M., Sugimoto, T., Takahashi, Y., Kaji, H., Kitazawa, R. & Chihara, K. (1998). Estrogen via the estrogen receptor blocks cAMP-mediated parathyroid hormone (PTH)-stimulated osteoclast formation. *J Bone Miner Res*, Vol.13, №5, (May 1998), pp. 854-862, ISSN 0884-0431

Kancheva, R., Sulkova, S., Svara, F., Hill, M., Kanchev, L. & Zofkova, I. (2008). Increase of nocturnal melatonin levels in hemodialyzed patients after parathyroidectomy – a pilot study. *Physiol Res*, Vol. 57, (Suppl. 1), (Feb 2008), pp. 181-185, ISSN 0862-8408.

Karasek, M., Szuflet, A., Chrzanowski, W., Zylinska, K. & Swietoslawski, J. (2002). Circadian serum melatonin profiles in patients suffering from chronic renal failure. *Neuro Endocrinol Lett,* Vol. 23, (Suppl 1), (Apr 2002), pp. 97-102, ISSN 0172-780X

Karasek, M., Szuflet, A., Chrzanowski, W., Zylinska, K. & Swietoslawski, J. (2005). Decreased melatonin nocturnal concentrations in hemodialyzed patients. *Neuro Endocrinol Lett*, Vol. 26, № 6 (Dec 2005), pp. 653-656, ISSN 0172-780X

Kenny, AM., Gallagher, JC., Prestwood, KM., Gruman, CA. & Raisz, LG. (1998). Bone density, bone turnover, and hormone levels in men over age 75. *J Gerontol A Biol Sci Med Sci*, Vol. 53, № 6, (Nov 1998), pp. 419-425, ISSN 1079-5006

Kiss, J., Banhegyi, D. & Scaba, G. (1969). Endocrine regulation of blood calcium level. II. Relationship between the pineal body and the parathyroid glands. (1969). *Acta Med Acad Sci Hungar*, Vol. 26, № 4, (Apr 1969), pp. 363-370, ISSN 0001-5989

Koch, BC., Nagtegaal, JE., Hagen, EC., Ter Wee, PM. & Kerkhof, GA. (2010b). Different melatonin rhythms and sleep-wake rhythms in patients on peritoneal dialysis, daytime hemodialysis and nocturnal hemodialysis. *Sleep Med*, Vol. 11, № 3, (Mar 2010), pp. 242-246, ISSN 1389-9457

Koch, BC., van der Putten, K., Van Someren, EJ., Wielders, J.P, Ter Wee, PM., Nagtegaal, JE. & Gaillard, CA. (2010a). Impairment of endogenous melatonin rhythm is related to the degree of chronic kidney disease (CREAM study). *Nephrol Dial Transplant*, Vol. 25, №2, (Feb 2010), pp. 513-519, ISSN 0931-0509

Koch, BC., Hagen, EC., Nagtegaal, JE., Boringa, JB., Kerkhof, GA. & Ter Wee, PM.(2009b). Effects of nocturnal hemodialysis on melatonin rhythm and sleep-wake behavior an uncontrolled trial. *Am J Kidney Dis*, Vol. 53, № 4, (Apr 2009), pp. 658-664, ISSN 0272-6386

Koch, BC., Nagtegaal, JE., Hagen, EC., van der Westerlaken, MM., Boringa, JB., Kerkhof, GA. & Ter Wee, PM. (2009a). The effects of melatonin on sleep-wake rhythm of daytime haemodialysis patients a randomized, placebo-controlled, cross-over study (EMSCAP study). *Br J Clin Pharmacol*, Vol. 67, № 1, (Jan 2009), pp. 68-75, ISSN 0306-5251

Komaba, H., & Fukagawa, M. (2010). FGF23-parathyroid interaction implications in chronic kidney disease. *Kidney Int*, Vol. 77, № 4, (Feb 2010), pp. 292-298, ISSN 0085-2538

Kovács, L., Szilágyi, G., Szabolcs, I. & Góth, M. (1994). The reaction of adenohypophysis hormones in primary hyperparathyroidism and after surgical treatment. *Acta Med Hung*, Vol. 50, № 1-2, (Feb 1994), pp. 15-21, ISSN 0236-5286

Kovanic, P. (1986). A new theoretical and algorithmic basis for estimation, identification and control. *Automatica*, Vol. 22, (1986), pp. 657-674, ISSN 0005-1098

Koyama, H., Nakade, O., Takada, Y., Kaku, T. & Lau, KH. (2002). Melatonin at pharmacologic doses increases bone mass by suppressing resorption through down-regulation of the RANKL-mediated osteoclast formation and activation. *J Bone Miner Res*, Vol. 17, № 7, (Jul 2002), pp. 1219-1229, ISSN 0884-0431

Krstic, R. (1966). The target method in the measurement of parathyroid cell activity after epiphysectomy. *Experientia*, Vol. 22, № 5, (May 1996), pp. 336-337, ISSN 0014-4754

Ladizesky, MG., Boggio, V., Albornoz, LE., Castrillon, PO., Mautalen, M. & Cardinali, DP. (2003). Melatonin increases oestradiol-induced bone formation in ovariectomized rats. *J Pineal Res* , Vol. 34, № 2, (Mar 2003), pp. 143-151, ISSN 0742-3098

Lamb, EJ., Vickery, S. & Ellis, AR. (2007). Parathyroid hormone, kidney disease, evidence and guidelines. *Ann Clin Biochem*, Vol. 44, № 1, (Jan 2007), pp. 1-4, ISSN 0004-5632

Leder, BZ., LeBlanc, KM., Schoenfeld, DA., Eastell, R. & Finkelstein, JS. (2003). Differential effects of androgens and estrogens on bone turnover in normal men. J *Clin Endocrinol Metab*, Vol. 88, №1, (Jan 2003), pp. 204-210, ISSN 0021-972X

Lindberg, MK., Vandenput, L., Movèrare Skrtic, S., Vanderschueren, D., Boonen, S., Bouillon, R. & Ohlsson, C. (2005). Androgens and the skeleton. *Minerva Endocrinol*, Vol. 30, № 1, (Mar 2005), pp. 15-25, ISSN 0391-1977

Liu, SZ., Tian, LF., Xu, P., Zhuang, GH., Zheng, F., Tian, J., Ning, QL., Zhu, BF., Lu, SM. & Yan, H. (2011.) Analysis of correlation between blood biochemical indicators and bone mineral density of post-menopausal women. *Mol Biol Rep*, Vol. 38, № 2, (Feb 2011), pp. 939-948, ISSN 0301-4851

Lüdemann, P., Zwernemann, S. & Lerchl, A. (2001). Clearance of melatonin and 6-sulfatoxymelatonin by hemodialysis in patients with end-stage renal disease. J Pineal Res, Vol. 31, № 3, (Oct 2001), pp. 222-227, ISSN 1600-079X

Malberti, F. (2010). Management of hyperphosphatemia in dialysis patients the role of phosphate binders. *G Ital Nefrol.*, Vol. 27, (Supp 52), (Nov-Dec, 2010), pp. 47-54, ISSN 0393-5590

Manolagas, SC. (2000) Birth and death of bone cells basic regulatory mechanisms and implications for the pathogenesis and treatment of osteoporosis. *Endocr Rev*,Vol. 21, №2, (Apr 2000), pp. 115-137, ISSN 0163-769X

Martin ,KJ. González, EA. (2011). Prevention and control of phosphate retention/hyperphosphatemia in CKD-MBD what is normal, when to start, and how to treat? *Clin J Am Soc Nephrol*, Vol. 6, (Feb 2011), pp. 440-446, ISSN, 1555-9041

Melhus, H., Michaëlsson, K., Holmberg, L., Wolk, A. & Ljunghall, S. (1999). Smoking, antioxidant vitamins, and the risk of hip fracture. *J Bone Miner Res.*, Vol. 14, № 1, (Jan 1999), pp. 129-135, ISSN 0884-0431

Molony, DA. & Stephens, BW. (2011). Dearrangements in phosphate metabolism in chronic kidney diseases/end stage renal disease therapeutic considerations. *Adv Chronic Kidney Dis*, Vol. 18, № 2, (Mar 2011), pp. 120-131, ISSN 1548-5595

Meloun, M., Militky, J., Hill, M. & Brereton, RG. (2002). Crucial problems in regression modeling and their solution. *Analyst*, Vol. 127, № 4, (Apr 2002), pp. 433-450, ISSN 0003-2654

Meloun, M., Hill, M., Militky, J. & Kupka, K. (2000). Transformation in the PC-aided biochemical data analysis. *Clin Chem Lab Med*, Vol. 38, № 6, (Jan 2000), pp. 553-559, ISSN 1434-6621

Miller, JE., Kovesdy, CP., Norris, KC., Mehrotra, R., Nissenson, AR., Kopple, JD. & Kalantar-Zadeh, K. (2010). Association of cumulatively low or high serum calcium levels with mortality in long-term hemodialysis patients. *Am J Nephrol*, Vol. 32, № 5, (Sep 2010), pp. 403-413, ISSN 0250-8095

Moe, SM., Drüeke, T., Lameire, N. & Eknoyan, G. (2007). Chronic kidney disease-mineral-bone disorder a new paradigm. *Adv Chronic Kidney Dis*, Vol. 14, № 1, (Jan 2007), pp. 3-12, ISSN 1548- 5595.

Monfort, M., Delanaye, P., Chapelle, JP. & Cavalier, E. (2008). Plasma calcium in haemodialysis patients total calcium or ionized calcium? Should we systematically provide a value of total corrected calcium on our protocols? *Ann Biol Clin (Paris)* , Vol. 66, № 5, (Sep-Oct 2008), pp. 573-576, ISSN 0003-3898

Morton, AR., Garland, JS. & Holden, RM. (2010). Is the calcium correct? Measuring serum calcium in dialysis patients. *Semin Dial*, Vol. 23, № 3, (May-Jun 2010), pp. 283-9, ISSN 0894-0959

Nakai, K., Komaba, H., & Fukagawa, M. (2010). New insights into the role of fibroblast growth factor 23 in chronic kidney disease. *Nephrol*, Vol. 23, № 6, (Nov-Dec 2010), pp. 619-625, ISSN 1121-8428

Nuti, R., Martini, G., Merlotti, D., De Paola, V., Valleggi, F. & Gennari, L. (2007). Bone metabolism in men and role of aromatase activity. *J Endocrinol Invest*, Vol. 30, (6 Suppl), pp. 18-23, ISSN 0391-4097

Ostrowska, Z., Ziora, K., Kos-Kudła, B., Swietochowska, E., Oświecimska, J., Dyduch, A., Wołkowska-Pokrywa, K. & Szapska, B. (2010). Melatonin, the RANKL/RANK/OPG system, and bone metabolism in girls with anorexia nervosa. *Endokrynol Pol*, Vol. 61, № 1, (Jan-Feb 2010), pp. 117-123, ISSN 0423-104X

Ostrowska, Z., Kos-Kudla, B., Nowak, M., Swietochowska, E., Marek, B., Gorski, J., Kajdaniuk, D. & Wolkowska, K. (2003b). The relationship between bone metabolism, melatonin and other hormones in sham-operated and pinealectomized rats. *Endocr Regul*, Vol. 37, № 4, (Dec 2003), pp. 211-224, ISSN 1210-0668

Ostrowska, Z., Kos-Kudla, B., Marek, B. & Kajdaniuk, D. (2003a). Influence of lighting conditions on daily rhythm of bone metabolism in rats and possible involvement of melatonin and other hormones in this process. *Endocr Regul*, Vol. 37, № 3, (Sep 2003), pp. 163-174, ISSN 1210-0668

Ostrowska, Z., Kos-Kudla, B., Swietochowska, E., Marek, B., Kajdaniuk, D. & Górski, J. (2001). Assessment of the relationship between dynamic pattern of nighttime levels of melatonin and chosen biochemical markers of bone metabolism in a rat model of postmenopausal osteoporosis. *Neuro Endocrinol Lett*, Vol. 22, № 2, (Apr 2001), pp. 129-136, ISSN 0172-780X

Panidis, D., Balaris, C., Farmakiotis, D., Rousso, D., Kourtis, A., Balaris, V., Katsikis, I., Zournatzi, V., & Diamanti-Kandarakis, E. (2005). Serum parathyroid hormone concentrations are increased in women with polycystic ovary syndrome. *Clin Chem*, Vol. 51, № 9, (Sep 2005), pp. 1691-1697, ISSN 0009- 9147

Pirklbauer, M. & Mayer, G. (2011). The exchangeable calcium pool physiology and pathophysiology in chronic kidney disease. *Nephrol Dial Transplant*, Vol.26, № 8, (Aug 2011), pp. 2438-2444, ISSN 0931-0509

Qunibi, WY. (2007). Cardiovascular calcification in nondialyzed patients with chronic kidney disease. *Semin Dial*, Vol. 20, № 2, (Mar-Apr 2007), pp. 134-138, ISSN 0894-0959

Raggi, P., Bommer, J., & Chertow, GM. (2004). Valvular calcification in hemodialysis patients randomized to calcium-based phosphorus binders or sevelamer. *J Heart Valve Dis*, Vol.13, № 1 (Jan 2004), pp. 134-141, ISSN 0966-8519

Riggs, BL., Khosla, S. & Melton, LJ. 3rd. (2002.) Sex steroids and the construction and conservation of the adult skeleton. *Endocr Rev*, Vol. 23, № 3, (Jun 2002), pp. 279-302, ISSN 0163-769X

Reiter, RJ., Paredes, SD., Manchester, LC. & Tan, DX. (2009). Reducing oxidative/nitrosative stress a newly-discovered genre for melatonin. *Crit Rev Biochem Mol Biol*, Vol. 44, № 4, (Jul-Aug 2009), pp. 175-200, ISSN 1040-9238

Reiter, RJ., Tan, DX., Manchester, LC. & Qi, W. (2001). Biochemical reactivity of melatonin with reactive oxygen and nitrogen species a review of the evidence. *Cell Biochem Biophys*, Vol. 34, № 2, (Mar 2001) pp. 237-256, ISSN 1085-9195

Rochira, V., Zirilli, L., Madeo, B., Aranda, C., Caffagni , G., Fabre, B., Montangero, VE., Roldan, EJ., Maffei, L. & Carani, C. (2007). Skeletal effects of long-term estrogen and testosterone replacement treatment in a man with congenital aromatase deficiency evidences of a priming effect of estrogen for sex steroids action on bone. *Bone*, Vol. 40, № 6, (Jun 2007), pp. 1662-1668, ISSN 8756-3282

Roth, JA., Kim, BG., Lin, WL. & Cho, MI. (1999) Melatonin promotes osteoblast differentiation and bone formation. *J Biol Chem*, Vol. 274, № 31, (Jul 1999), pp. 22041-22047, ISSN 0021-9258

Rudser, KD., de Boer, IH., Dooley, A., Young, B. & Kestenbaum, B. (2007). Fracture risk after parathyroidectomy among chronic hemodialysis patients. *J Am Soc Nephrol*, Vol. 18, № 8, (Aug 2007), pp. 2401-2407, ISSN 1555-9041

Salamano, G., Isaia, GC., Pecchio, F., Appendino, S., Mussetta, M. & Molinatti, GM. (1990). Effect on phospho-calcium metabolism of testosterone administration in hypogonadal males. *Arch Ital Urol Nefrol Androl*, Vol. 62, № 1, (Mar 1990), pp. 149-153, ISSN 1120-8538

Sánchez-Barceló, EJ., Mediavilla, MD., Tan, DX. & Reiter, RJ. (2010). Scientific basis for the potential use of melatonin in bone diseases osteoporosis and adolescent idiopathic scoliosis. *J Osteoporos*, Vol. 2010, doi: 10.4061/2010/830231, ISSN 2090-8059

Sandyk, R., Anastasiadis, PG., Anninos, PA. & Tsagas, N. (1992). Is postmenopausal osteoporosis related to pineal gland functions? *Int J Neurosci*, Vol. 62, № 3-4, (Feb 1992), pp. 215-225, ISSN 0020-7454

Sawaya, BP., Monier-Faugere, MC., Ratanapanichkich, P., Butros, R., Wedlund, PJ. & Fanti, P. (2002). Racial differences in parathyroid hormone levels in patients with secondary hyperparathyroidism. *Clin Nephrol*, Vol. 57, № 1, (Jan 2002), pp. 51-55, ISSN 0301-0430

Shoumura, S., Chen, H., Emura, S., Utsumi, M., Hayakawa, D., Yamahira, T., Terasawa, K., Tamada, A., Arakawa, M. & Isono H. (1992). An in vitro study on the effects of melatonin on the ultrastructure of the hamster parathyroid gland. *Histol Histopathol*, Vol. 7, № 4, (Oct 1992), pp. 715-718, ISSN 0213-3911

Suzuki, N. & Hattori, A. (2002). Melatonin suppresses osteoclastic and osteoblastic activities in the scales of goldfish. *J Pineal Res*, Vol. 33, № 4, (Nov 2002), pp. 253-258, ISSN 0742-3098

Tan, DX., Manchester, LC., Reiter, RJ., Qi, WB., Zhang, M., Weintraub, ST., Cabrera, J., Sainz, RM. & Mayo, JC. (1999). Identification of highly elevated levels of melatonin in bone marrow its origin and significance. *Biochem Biophys Acta*, Vol. 1472, № 1-2 (Oct 1999), pp. 206-214, ISSN 0006-3002

Tominaga, Y., Uchida, K., Haba, T., Katayama, A., Sato, T., Hibi, Y., Numano, M., Tanaka, Y., Inagaki, H., Watanabe, I., Hachisuka, T. & Takagi, H. (2001). More than 1,000 cases of total parathyroidectomy with forearm autograft for renal hyperparathyroidism. *Am J Kidney Dis*, Vol. 38, № 4, (Suppl. 1), (Oct 2001), pp. 168-171, ISSN 0272-6386

Vanderschueren, D., Vandenput, L., Boonen, S., Lindberg, MK., Bouillon, R. & Ohlsson, C. (2004). Androgens and bone. *Endocr Rev*, Vol. 25, № 3 (Jun 2004), pp. 389-425, ISSN 0163- 769X

Vaziri, ND., Oveisi, F., Wierszbiezki, M., Shaw, V. & Sporty, LD. (1993). Serum melatonin and 6-sulfatoxymelatonin in end-stage renal disease effect of hemodialysis. *Artif Organs*, Vol. 17, № 9, (Sep 1993), pp. 764-9, ISSN 0160-564X

Viljoen, M., Steyn, ME., van Rensburg, BW. & Reinach, SG. (1992). Melatonin in chronic renal failure. *Nephron*, Vol. 60, № 2,(Jan 1992), pp. 138-143, ISSN 0028-2766

Wikner, J., Wetterberg, L. & Röjdmark, S. (1997). Does hypercalcaemia or calcium antagonism affect human melatonin secretion or renal excretion? *Eur J Clin Invest*, Vol. 27, № 5 (May 1997), pp. 374-379, ISSN 0014-2972

Wiren, KM., Semirale, AA., Zhang, XW., Woo, A., Tommasini, SM., Price, C., Schaffler, MB. & Jepsen, KJ. (2008). Targeting of androgen receptor in bone reveals a lack of androgen anabolic action and inhibition of osteogenesis a model for compartment-specific androgen action in the skeleton. *Bone*, Vol. 43, № 3 (Sep 2008), pp. 440-441, ISSN 8756- 3282

Wolden-Hanson, T., Mitton, DR., McCants, RL., Yellon, SM., Wilkinson, CW., Matsumoto, AM. & Rasmussen, DD. (2000). Daily melatonin administration to middle-aged male rats suppresses body weight, intraabdominal adiposity, and plasma leptin and insulin independent of food intake and total body fat. *Endocrinology*, Vol. 141, № 2, (Feb 2000), pp. 487-497, ISSN 0013-7227

Yano, S., Sugimoto, T., Tsukamoto, T., Yamaguchi, T., Hattori, T., Sekita, KI., Kaji, H., Hattori, S., Kobayashi, A. & Chihara, K. (2003). Effect of parathyroidectomy on bone mineral density in hemodialysis patients with secondary hyperparathyroidism possible usefulness of preoperative determination of parathyroid hormone level for prediction of bone regain. *Horm Metab Res*, Vol. 35, №4 , (Jan 2003), pp. 259-264, ISSN 0018-5043

Young, EW., Albert, JM., Satayathum, S., Goodkin, DA., Pisoni. RL., Akiba, T., Akizawa, T., Kurokawa, K., Bommer, J., Piera, L. & Port, FK. (2005). Predictors and consequences of altered mineral metabolism the dialysis autcomes and practice patterns study. *Kidney Int*, Vol. 67, № 3, (Mar 2005), pp. 1179-1187, ISSN 0085-2538

Zaminy, A., Barbarestani, M., Hedayatpour, A., Mahmoudi, R. & Farzaneh Nejad, A. (2008). Osteogenic differentiation of rat mesenchymal stem cells from adipose tissue in comparison with bone marrow mesenchymal stem cells melatonin as a differentiation factor. *Iran Biomed J*, Vol. 12, № 3, (Jul 2008), pp. 133-141, ISSN 1028-852X

Zirilli, L., Rochira, V., Diazzi, C., Caffagni, G. & Carani, C. (2008). Human models of aromatase deficiency. *J Steroid Biochem Mol Biol*, Vol. 109, № 3-5, (Apr 2008), pp. 212-218, ISSN 0960-0760

Zofkova, I., Röjdmark, S. & Kancheva, RL. (1993). Does estrogen replacement therapy influence parathyroid hormone responsiveness to exogenous hypercalcemia in postmenopausal women? *J Endocrinol Invest*, Vol. 16, № 5 (May 1993), pp. 323-327, ISSN 0391-4097

Zofkova, I., Röjdmark, S. & Kancheva, RL. (1994). Stanazolol--an anabolic steroid that does not influence parathyroid hormone response to hypercalcemia in postmenopausal women. *Calcif Tissue Int*, Vol. 54, № 6, (Jun 1994), pp. 521-522, ISSN 0171-967X

Zofkova, I., Sotorník, I., & Kancheva, RL. (1996). Adenohypophyseal-gonadal dysfunction in male haemodialyzed patients before and after subtotal parathyroidectomy. *Nephron*, Vol. 74, №3, (Mar 1996), pp. 536-540, ISSN 0028-2766